S0-BAA-959

Planet Widow

A Mother's Story of Navigating a Suddenly

Unrecognizable World

Gloria Lenhart

SEAL PRESS

Planet Widow
A Mother's Story of Navigating a Suddenly Unrecognizable World

Copyright © 2006 by Gloria Lenhart

Some photos and illustrations are used by permission and are the property of the original copyright owners.

Photo used on page vi, 55, and 249: Astronomy Digital Vision

Published by
Seal Press
An Imprint of Avalon Publishing Group, Incorporated
1400 65th Street, Suite 250
Emeryville, CA 94608

AVALON
publishing group incorporated

All rights reserved. No part of this book may be reproduced or transmitted in any form without written permission from the publisher, except by reviewers who may quote brief excerpts in connection with a review.

ISBN-10 1-58005-168-5
ISBN-13 978-1-58005-168-2

9 8 7 6 5 4 3 2 1

Library of Congress Cataloging-in-Publication Data
Lenhart, Gloria.
 Planet widow : a mother's story of navigating a suddenly unrecognizable world / Gloria Lenhart.
 p. cm.
 ISBN-13: 978-1-58005-168-2
 ISBN-10: 1-58005-168-5
 1. Widowhood. 2. Adjustment (Psychology) 3. Grief. 4. Widowhood—Psychological aspects. I. Title.
HQ1058.L46 2006
155.9'37—dc22
 2005030344

Cover and interior design by Domini Dragoone
Printed in the United States of America by Worzalla
Distributed by Publishers Group West

For my sons
Nikolaus and Matthew
Papa would be so proud of you

Contents

PART 3 The Beginning

PART 1 The End

Nothing to Do but Wait

chapter one

There are ordinary days and there are extraordinary days. The ordinary days make up the bulk of our lives; the extraordinary days provide the punctuation. Some extraordinary days we hope for, wait for, plan for. Some come on us suddenly, unexpectedly, unasked. They are the bends in the road that lead us in unexpected directions and take us to unforeseen destinations, to worlds we didn't even know were there.

Today is Thursday. It is not an ordinary day. Today I will bury my husband.

Nick died on Saturday, a day that began as ordinary and then went very wrong. On Saturday, there were flashing lights, wailing sirens, and doctors in white shirts. Today, there will be candles, organ music, and a priest in purple vestments.

My black wool suit and red silk blouse are pressed and ready.

"You're not going to wear red to the funeral," my mother said last night, forgetting as she often does that I'm forty-two years old, not twelve.

My sister silenced her quickly. "For God's sake, Mother, her husband dropped dead. The last thing she needs from us right now is fashion advice."

Nick liked me in red. I was wearing red the day I met him. I want to wear red to say goodbye.

I want Nick's funeral to be just right. I want everything to be just the way Nick would have wanted it. I want to make him proud.

Nick's cousin Tom drove down from Sacramento to help me with the arrangements. Tom and Nick were like brothers, maybe closer than brothers. Nick was older by a few years, and even as adults, Tom looked up to him. Tom is an emergency room nurse, so he's used to dealing with life and death. I know he is someone I can count on.

Tom helped me pick the suit Nick will wear today, the one he will be buried in. Nick liked to dress well—not to impress anyone but because he loved nice clothes in the same way he appreciated anything that displayed craftsmanship. His job as manager of distribution and imports for Mervyn's, a department store chain, required a wardrobe of suits and ties and gave him the opportunity to shop in cities throughout the world. His suits were custom made in London and Hong Kong. He bought his shoes in Brazil. He liked Italian silk ties.

"I don't even own a suit," Tom said, looking down the line of neatly pressed jackets, knife-edged slacks, and the crisp procession of starched shirts that hung on Nick's side of our walk-in closet.

"I'm sorry that none of these fit you," I said, running my hand down a soft wool sleeve. Tom is tall, lean, blond; Nick was shorter, stocky, and dark.

Tom and I took a long time selecting the right suit for Nick. I wanted to make just the right choice. I tried to think of what Nick would want to wear. We quickly eliminated the European cuts (too trendy), the lightweight summer tans (wrong season), and anything black (too somber). "How about the tuxedo?" Tom asked.

"He's only worn it twice," I said. "He bought it for our wedding, and then he wore it one year on Halloween."

We finally agreed on the blue wool double-breasted. Nick seldom wore it because he thought it made him look heavy. But it was dark and conservative and seemed to fit the occasion.

"The guy at the funeral home said you could send a pair of shoes along if you want," Tom said. Without hesitation, I pulled out Nick's favorite cowboy boots. He had had them custom made in Texas. "They don't really go with the suit," Tom said, but I insisted.

Socks and underwear probably weren't necessary, but I packed some anyway. I hesitated in front of Nick's tie rack. "I think the boys should pick the tie," I said.

Tom looked over the lineup of ties progressing from blues to greens to yellows to reds. "Maybe you should narrow down the selection for them."

I eliminated the ones with cartoon characters, the hunting and fishing themes, the various holiday motifs, and the wildest colors and patterns. Presenting my two sons with three conservative choices, I could see by their faces that they were less than enthused.

"Are you sure these are Papa's?" sixteen-year-old Nikolaus asked. "I've never seen them before."

"Papa wouldn't wear those ties," six-year-old Matthew agreed. "They're boring."

We returned to the tie rack and debated the merits and drawbacks of a dozen other choices. Finally, we agreed on the tie

Matthew had bought Nick last Father's Day. He had used his own money and picked it out himself. It was a pulsating pattern of yellow, green, and blue. "Papa loves this tie," Matthew insisted.

"I could get rid of the rest of these clothes for you," Tom said.

"There'll be time for that later," I said. I carefully readjusted the remaining suits.

The suits that Nikolaus and Matthew will wear today hang on my side of the closet. Nikolaus's is nearly man-sized, while Matthew's is smaller. Both are brand new. I had to take each boy shopping for funeral-appropriate clothes.

The salesgirl at the Men's Wearhouse had looked at Nikolaus admiringly as he shrugged into a jacket and turned for our assessment. "Your date will be very impressed," she cooed. Nikolaus and I looked at her blankly, wondering if we should tell her what the suit was really for.

She eyed the plain white shirt and black tie that I had selected with obvious distaste. "Collarless shirts are really cool," she suggested, pointedly turning her back on me and focusing on Nikolaus, "Or a sweater would be totally hip." Nikolaus was giving me desperate *Help me* looks over her shoulder.

"This will do for now," I said, firmly placing my credit card on top of my totally unhip selections.

"You can always try different looks with that suit later," the salesgirl told Nikolaus, brushing imaginary lint off his sweater. I was thinking of burning the suit after the funeral, but I kept that to myself.

I take both boys' suits out of the closet now and lay each carefully across the foot of my bed. It's a little after four in the morning, but I know I won't sleep. I might as well get dressed. It takes only a few minutes to slip on my skirt and tuck in my blouse. I don't bother with makeup. Even the little makeup I normally wear feels garish, a painted-on cheerfulness I can't maintain. I soak my wedding ring in a jar of jewelry cleaner and then scrub the backsides of the diamond gently with a tiny brush. I slip it on, and its small, familiar weight on my left hand is a comfort. It seems to bring me back into balance.

I open a dresser drawer and withdraw a small, flat box. Inside, a gold cross is suspended on a delicate chain. My grandmother gave me this cross on my Confirmation Day. I've worn it on happier days—the day I was married, the day Matthew was christened. I wore it on those days to ensure blessing and to protect my happiness. Today, I see the cross as what it really is: a symbol of suffering.

Time is extraordinarily slow, each minute a ponderous weight. Since the day Nick died, I have been climbing an endless ladder, intently focused on each rung, afraid that any misstep may plunge me down into some great void. I haven't thought any further ahead than this day, Thursday, the day I will lay Nick to rest. Maybe after today, I will be able to rest, too. I haven't slept at all. Each night, I climb the stairs to my room, exhausted. Each night, I lie in our bed, alone, my thoughts racing: flower arrangements, memorial speeches, thank you notes, money, bills. Can I afford to stay in this house? How much chicken salad should I order? Should I talk to a lawyer? There is so much to do now, so much to decide. While everyone else sleeps, I plan, worry, and wait.

As I lie alone in bed each night, I ache to see sign—a flash, a twinkle—something that tells me that I am not alone. I see nothing. I wait to feel a warm breeze, a cold sweat, a wave of peacefulness that would indicate that Nick is with me. I feel nothing. Every night since Nick died, I lie still, alone, and wait as the blackness of the night slowly turns to the gray of morning.

On this morning, though, I cannot lie still. I remember the day Nick and I got married. I couldn't sleep that day, either. I was up early and fully dressed by ten in the morning, although the wedding wouldn't be until one o'clock. While my sisters were still fussing with their hair and makeup, I was all ready, standing by the window of my room, waiting. Do all brides carry the worry, however small, that their grooms will have a last-minute change of heart? Suddenly, a bright-red toy jeep sped across the sidewalk under my window. It was followed by Nick and Nikolaus, dressed in matching black tuxedos. Nikolaus, then just seven years old, ran after the jeep, joyously clutching a remote-control device. Nick looked up through the tree and saw me standing at the window. My smile said, "I'm ready." His smile answered, "I can't wait."

Now I sit on the edge of our bed, careful not to wrinkle my skirt, and look out a different window. The world outside is dark and empty. There is plenty of time. All the arrangements are set. The limo won't come for us until nine. There is nothing to do now but wait.

Not a Trace

chapter two

There is a fundamental difference between women who are widows and women who are not widows. Women who are not widows will recall a time when their husbands experienced chest pains, or were almost in a car accident, or had some medical problem that turned out to be not so serious after all, and they will always say, "I thought for sure he was going to die." Widows, on the other hand, will always say, "I never thought that he was going to die." Sometimes I think that the reason Nick died is because I never thought he would.

Widows are very specific about death. We remember the details. Ask us when our husbands died and we won't say, "Last month" or "At the end of April." We'll say April 16, or November 28, or June 6. Nick died on February 7. It was a Saturday. No one knows exactly what time he died. It happened somewhere on the street, a few blocks from our house. By the time I arrived, he had already been moved into the ambulance. If he had final words, there was no one there to hear them. In the middle of an otherwise predictable suburban Saturday morning, he died instantly and alone.

A neighbor drove by and saw him lying on the sidewalk. It was raining, but she stopped her car and got out, and saw right away that something was terribly wrong. She searched for Nick's pulse. She tried to force her breath into his mouth. She banged on his chest. While all this was happening, I was catching up on paperwork in my upstairs office. I earn a living by writing marketing plans, brochures, websites, and training programs for companies like Charles Schwab and Wells Fargo. Being able to work at home is convenient, but the downside is that it's tough to get away from your office. That morning, when my neighbor rushed over to tell me that Nick was in an ambulance down the street, I was still in my bathrobe, even though it was almost noon. The kids were watching Saturday morning cartoons. None of us could say exactly when Nick had left the house. He hadn't told us he was leaving; he hadn't said goodbye.

The autopsy report shows that there were cuts on Nick's nose and forehead. There were none on his hands, his elbows, or his knees. Tom says that means Nick literally dropped dead. Tom can translate medical terms and read between the lines: Tom says that if Nick had scraped his knees or his hands, that would have meant that he felt it coming and had time to feel pain or fear. Instead, Nick fell flat on his face. Tom says he probably never knew what hit him.

By the time I got there, Nick was in the ambulance, and two medics were on either side of him, pounding and pumping. There were lots of tubes and knobs and needles. There was no room for me inside the ambulance, so I stood outside. I remember the pattern on the soles of Nick's shoes, his hand hanging limply off the gurney, a sudden rain shower pelting on my head and dribbling down my back.

Someone offered to drive me to the hospital, but I said I had to go back to the house first and tell the kids what was happening. I told the kids that I was going to the hospital with Papa, and I promised to call them with any news. They looked as scared as I felt.

"Everything is going to be alright," I promised them. I wasn't lying—I really believed my own words.

Nick's glasses lay on the table by the front door. He didn't like to wear them while running. He'll need those, I thought. I didn't want to scratch or break them by putting them in my pocket, so I held them in my hands.

On the way to the hospital, I remember thinking, *They'll be able to fix him. He'll be okay.*

My neighbor dropped me off in front of the emergency entrance. "Are you sure you'll be alright?" he asked. "Sure, sure," I said. The fact that Nick might already be dead never crossed my mind. I never thought he would die.

—⚡—

Nick knew all about hospitals. He himself had never been sick, but he spent a lot of time in hospitals with his first wife, Rachael.

Rachael had been diagnosed with Type I diabetes—"juvenile diabetes," they used to call it—when she was fourteen. At twenty-four, she married Nick. Though she knew it was risky, Rachael was determined to have a child. She had five miscarriages in four years before delivering a tiny, two-pound boy, eight weeks premature. They named him Nikolaus.

Two-pound babies have about a 90 percent chance of survival today, but back then, Nikolaus's chances were fifty-fifty. He was born on the Fourth of July, but he didn't leave the hospital until just before Christmas.

After giving birth, Rachael's diabetes spiraled out of control. Her circulation slowed. The toes on her right foot had to be amputated, and then they took the rest of her leg. When her kidneys failed, she was on dialysis for months. She had one kidney transplant, and when that failed, she had another. It became clear to everyone but Nick that Rachael was fighting a losing battle. Nick did everything he could to save her, but she died in a San Francisco hospital just short of her thirty-third birthday.

Nick never said much about how difficult that time was for him, coping with both a premature baby and a seriously ill wife. He just did it. Nick consulted with doctors, filed medical forms, investigated treatments and procedures, cleaned Rachael's wounds, kept track of her medication, rallied her spirits. Now it was going to be up to me to do the same thing for Nick. As I waited my turn at the emergency room desk, I felt like I was ready.

—ᴠᴠ—

A nurse escorted me from the emergency room entrance down a corridor to a small, windowless room. I wondered where Nick was and why they hadn't brought me right in to see him. I thought maybe the doctors were working on him, or maybe he was in surgery. I stood and waited, still holding Nick's glasses in my hand.

An eternity passed. Then, a man in a white jacket came in and introduced himself. Dr. Someone. He was very particular about confirming who I was.

"I have my husband's glasses," I said, as if this were positive identification. "He probably needs them."

The doctor looked at the glasses in my hand for what seemed like a long time. "Your husband is dead," he said finally. "I'm sorry." Simple and direct. Two pieces of information, separate but related. Your husband is dead. I'm sorry.

"What happened?" I asked.

The doctor looked away. "We don't know yet," he answered. I wondered how he got selected to tell me the news. He was probably wondering the same thing.

"Can I see him?"

I put Nick's glasses in my pocket and followed the doctor's white back down the hall. My legs were numb.

I guess I expected to find Nick laid out on his back, eyes closed, hands folded across his chest. That's how I expected the dead to look. But Nick didn't look that way. He was sprawled on a table in the middle of a big, empty room. He lay like a child who had fallen asleep on his mother's shoulder and had been gently put down, arms flung across the table, shoes still on. His head was turned toward the door, and there was a plastic tube in his mouth. His eyes were half open. Relief flooded through me when I saw him. My first thought was, *They got it wrong.*

I ran to his side and picked up his hand. It was surprisingly cold and heavy. Up close, his skin was blue-white. I whispered his name. His eyes were empty, his face chiseled and perfectly still.

In that moment, I knew that he was gone—completely and irretrievably gone.

I did not turn away from him—there was no reason to. This was not a grisly or horrific death. Only his heart had betrayed him, quietly and bloodlessly. I stood there, awed by the incredible audacity of death to take someone away so easily, so quickly, and leave behind a perfectly flawless representation of a person who is clearly no longer there. I don't believe that I had ever felt so totally alone.

I would have sat there and held Nick's hand forever, but after a while, a nurse came and led me back through halls of living, bleeding people. The air felt thick, heavy, and hard to breathe. The lights seemed very bright. I tried to think of what to do next.

"Do you want to call someone?" the nurse asked.

That seemed like a good idea. I tried to think of someone to call. The kids? No. Better to get home and tell them in person. My family? They were all on the other side of the country. What good would it do to call them now, from here? Nick's family? There were only his mother and his cousins. Tom lived two hours away; there was not much point in calling him. The thought of telling Nick's mother that her only son was dead was something I desperately wanted to put off. It was also something I knew I couldn't do over the phone.

I was cold now, freezing, but my back was dripping with sweat. *I have to get out of here,* I thought. *I have to get home.* I was trying desperately to think, forcing myself not to panic.

The nurse gave me a phone book, but I couldn't remember any of my friends' names. I tried to look up Nick's cousin Tina, who lives about twenty minutes away, the closest relative. I couldn't remember the order of the alphabet. I flipped through the pages, hoping to stumble on the Ts. The small type swam and danced. "I think I need help," I said to the nurse.

It took Tina over an hour to arrive; she got lost on the way. I sat in the waiting room, my mind numb. I took Nick's glasses out of my pocket and held them in my lap. After a while, a nurse noticed I was still there, sitting quietly among the sick and bleeding. She led me back to the concrete cube she called the Quiet Room. I perched on the plastic couch and stared at the celebrity faces smiling up at me from the magazine rack. By the time Tina arrived at the emergency room desk, the nurse who had helped me was busy with another emergency. No one there knew who or where I was.

I don't remember the drive home. I was worried that I hadn't called the boys, as I had promised, but I think bad news is better told in person. They ran into the hall to meet me when I walked in. "What happened?" Nikolaus asked. Matthew looked very frightened.

"Papa had a heart attack," I said. "I don't know exactly what happened or why, but he died." I suddenly realized that was the sum total of information I had.

I don't know what reaction I had expected them to have, but I guess I didn't expect them to be so calm. They were standing so still that I wondered if they had heard me. I thought I'd better tell them again. "When I got to the hospital, he was already dead," I said.

Nikolaus said, "Did you see him?"

"Yes. He looked . . ." I struggled for a word. Blue? Cold? Incredibly beautiful? "Peaceful," I said.

They both nodded. This seemed to satisfy them, to make sense. We stood looking at each other for a few moments, none of us knowing what to say. I remember thinking that the crying would come later. Right now, there seemed to be too much to do. "What should we do now?" Nikolaus asked.

"We need to tell Oma." Oma is the German word for grandmother. It's what the kids call Nick's mother.

"She'll be sad," Matthew said solemnly.

"We'll all be sad now," I told him.

I remember wanting to hug them both and to hold on to them as tightly as I could. I wish I had. But I was afraid that I'd break down, and I thought that if I broke down, it would scare the kids even more. They were both standing there stoically—one so small, one almost grown—waiting for whatever came next. As absurd as it sounds, I wanted them to feel that everything was going to be fine. I really wish that I had showed them that it was okay to be scared, that it was okay to cry. Instead, I told them that they should go play video games while I talked to Tina. "I have to figure out how to tell Oma," I told them.

The boys reluctantly climbed the stairs, as Tina and I slumped over to the kitchen table.

"I'm afraid to tell Elisabeth that her son is dead," I told Tina. "I'm afraid that she will fall apart."

My mother-in-law, Elisabeth, has led a life full of horrific events. She was a young girl in Yugoslavia when her mother died of cancer. Elisabeth dropped out of school to help raise her brothers and sisters. She married a soldier when she was still in her teens. Shortly after their daughter was born, her husband was killed in combat. Then the village where they lived came under fire in one of the many upheavals that has rocked Yugoslavia over the years. Elisabeth's family was forced to flee because they were of German descent. Fearing for her daughter's safety, she let her be adopted by a local Yugoslavian family who agreed to keep the child safe by pretending she was their own child. Elisabeth promised the adopting family that she would never contact the girl, a promise she kept until the 1980s when she found her daughter and helped her resettle in Germany during yet another Yugoslavian war.

After leaving her daughter, Elisabeth relocated to a small Yugoslavian village where she married her second husband, Nick's father. Nick was only a few months old when the family had an opportunity to relocate to Germany. They had to leave everything behind. Elisabeth has often told me of their long trip to Germany: crowded trains, devising diapers out of used clothing found in donation piles, weeks in a refugee camp until they found housing and jobs. Six years later, the family was settled in Germany with an apartment and jobs when they got permission to emigrate to the United States. Again, they left everything and went.

"My Aunt Elisabeth is tougher than you think," Tina said. "Remember, she's lost her mother, and her father and brother were shot to death in front of her. And she's buried two husbands."

"This is different," I said. "This is her son."

"I'll be there with you," Tina said.

"I don't want the kids there. She can be very dramatic. If she starts screaming or crying, they won't know what to do. I don't want them to see that."

Tina's husband had gone to pick up their two boys. Tina called him and asked that he bring their kids back to our house and wait with Matthew and Nikolaus until Tina and I got back from Elisabeth's house.

—⁓—

Elisabeth knew something was wrong the minute she saw us on her porch. I told her to sit down. I told her what happened. I told her that Nick was dead. She remained very quiet.

She sat so still for so long that I began to wonder if she had understood what I had said. Although Elisabeth had lived in the United States for over forty years, she still struggled a bit with the English language. She spoke and understood everyday English well enough, but I noticed that when she was sick or upset, she seemed more comfortable with the German or Croatian she learned as a young girl. I wasn't sure if she didn't understand what I said, or if she, like the kids, had to hear the unthinkable news twice before the meaning of the words could sink in. I asked Tina to repeat the news in German. Then, Elisabeth spoke.

"I don't believe it," she repeated again and again, although I knew that she did believe it.

"It's true," I said.

There was no crying, no screaming, no hysterics. In fact, it seemed to me that a preternatural quiet surrounded us, dampening the scrape of chairs on the floor and fading the traffic noise from the street. I helped Elisabeth pack a suitcase and lock up her house. We picked up fast food for the kids. Standing in line at McDonald's, I looked at all the other families eating their dinners, on their way to or from the movies or the mall. I felt like I was in a nightmare.

When we got back to the house, there were seventeen messages on the answering machine, all words of sympathy from neighbors who had heard the news. I thought about the small crowd that had been huddled behind the ambulance. While I was still hoping for the best, they all knew that he was already gone.

Nikolaus took charge of the kids, shepherding them upstairs to watch TV while the adults sat around the kitchen table: me, Elisabeth, Tina, and her husband. We tried to think of what we needed to do. Something would be suggested, someone would attend to it, and then we'd think of something else.

"You should call your mother," someone said, and I did.

"You should call Father Bob," someone suggested, and I did that, too.

I called the funeral home, my sisters, and Nick's boss. We made and drank endless pots of tea. By ten o'clock, when we couldn't think of anything else to do, Tina said, "We should be going home."

After Tina and her husband left, I helped Matthew get into his pajamas. We are not big on prayer, but we say grace before dinner and prayers before bed. Tonight, it seemed like a good idea for all of us to pray together. I tucked Matthew in, and then Nikolaus, Elisabeth, and I sat on the bed and prayed with him.

Now I lay me down to sleep, I pray the Lord my soul to keep. Guide me through the starry night, wake me with the sunshine bright. Amen.

The sun would not be shining for us tomorrow, or the next day, or the next. Matthew ended his prayer with, "Please God, bless Papa, wherever he is."

I locked the house and turned off the downstairs lights. Elisabeth went into the guest room and closed the door. I climbed the stairs to bed. I lay on Nick's side and buried my face in his pillow. The sheets felt cool and smelled clean. There were no reminders, no traces of Nick there. I wondered if I should cry. I turned over and stared up into the darkness and waited. I did not sleep.

What Would Jackie Do?

chapter three

Up until the 1940s, people generally died at home. A professional undertaker would be called in to "undertake" the preparation of the remains, order the coffin or casket, and coordinate the burial. Funerals were usually held in homes. The family would lay their loved one out in the "parlor," the formal room in the front of the house used to receive guests, then sit with the body day and night for two or three days while visitors came to pay their respects. Neighbors would bring food to sustain the family and flowers to lift their spirits. Death was part of the fabric of life.

At the end of World War I, a leading women's magazine promoted the transformation of the front parlor into what they renamed the "living room." As more and more people began to die in hospitals rather than at home, it became common for families to hold the funeral outside the home in funeral parlors. The funeral business is now a $25 billion industry. In 1998, the typical American funeral cost about $8,000.

Embalming dates back to the Egyptians, who refined the art for religious purposes. During the Civil War, embalming was commonly done for sanitation. Lincoln's funeral was a turning point in the popularity of the practice of applying cosmetics to the dead. A staff of embalmers accompanied the president on his final journey, a train ride from Washington D.C. to his hometown of Springfield, Illinois, that included stops in thirteen cities. Newspaper accounts remarked favorably on his appearance, and an estimated one million people lined the train tracks to view his body. This elaborate and dramatic farewell increased the acceptance of embalming for cosmetic purposes and it became established as the custom, particularly among Christians.

Lincoln's funeral was not the last time the death of a public figure has had a dramatic effect on burial customs. I am just old enough to remember the funeral of President John F. Kennedy. In November 1963, I was an impressionable eight-year-old, snowed in with my brother and sisters in suburban New Jersey, devouring every minute of the televised coverage. The horses, the music, John John's salute, the eternal flame. And Jackie, the ultimate widow: Ill-fated but courageous. Shrouded but capable. Architect of her husband's legacy. Protector of her children. Now, preparing for my own husband's funeral, I decided I could count on Jackie to help me through.

This morning, at 8:30 AM, a limo pulls into the driveway. A black limo. A long, black stretch limo, not the towncar limo I had ordered.

"We don't usually do limos," the funeral director had said on Monday, when Tom and I had gone to make the arrangements. "Usually people prefer to drive themselves."

"I can drive some people," Tom whispered to me, "and my parents can take some."

"I appreciate that," I whispered back, "but that won't be enough. My whole family is coming, a total of eleven people. I'm not driving, I'm not renting a bus, and I'm not up to arranging carpools." My inability to sleep had made me irritable, but it had also provided plenty of uninterrupted hours to plan the funeral in my head. I knew what I wanted, what Nick would have wanted. I needed this service to be perfect.

I turned back to the funeral director. "We'll need three limos."

The funeral director looked frightened. "I'm sure you won't need more than one." He gave me a pleading look. "It can get awfully expensive."

I tried to unclench my jaw. "I don't care what it costs. We cannot cram eleven people into one limo." At that point, I didn't care if it took me the rest of my life to pay it off. I wanted Nick to have a decent burial, and I was determined to give it to him.

Small beads of sweat shimmered on the funeral director's forehead. "I may be able to find two limos."

I was firm. "We will definitely need three. Send one to my home. Two more will be needed at the hotel for my family."

"How many people will be at the hotel?" The funeral director's voice was a squeak.

I knew what he was thinking, and I knew I had to head him off at the pass. "Seven in all. My two uncles and my mother are well past seventy and not all that spry. One of my sisters is seven months pregnant, and the other has multiple sclerosis. Any one of them may have to leave the service early, which would leave everyone else stranded or crammed into the other limo with us." I took a deep breath and turned on my Jackie charm. Jackie had arranged horse-drawn carriages, honor guards, and full network coverage. I forced a smile. "I'm sure that between now and Thursday, you can find three discreet, business-style limos somewhere in the San Francisco Bay Area."

"I'll make some calls," he said.

What Would Jackie Do?

—⟋⟍⟍—

On the morning of the funeral, all I know is that there is at least one black limo, although it is approximately the length of a football field. I decide to remain calm about the size and arrival of the other cars, which I hope are showing up at the hotel right now. I have done all I can, and it is time to go.

Elisabeth has been staying with us since Nick died. This morning, she helps me get the boys dressed and ready to go. No one has much appetite for breakfast. I tuck a bag of fruit, granola bars, and chocolate in the back of the limo in case we get hungry later. At least the unwanted limo comes complete with a fully stocked bar. I think about plying Elisabeth with a strong drink, but she appears calm enough. Besides, I'm afraid the interaction of alcohol and her medication could cause problems I don't need. I'm afraid to drink. I don't want to show up at the funeral a bit tipsy and have everyone think I can't cope. I need to keep my wits about me.

It only takes a half an hour to get to the church, and the service won't start for another two, but the limo idling outside is reason enough to be on our way. I have been dreading this day, and now I'm anxious to get on with it. The service will last no more than an hour. Father Bob told us we have to be out of the church no later than noon, at which time the kids at the Catholic school across the street will let out for lunch.

"It's upsetting for the children to see the caskets carried out of the church three or four times a week," the priest explained. When I was in Catholic school, no one shielded us from death. In fact, in the upper grades, we sang at about two funerals a month as part of the choir group. We didn't know any of the people whose services we sang for. They were faceless, nameless, interchangeable old people who had probably died in their sleep. Their funerals were all the same. First, a smattering of steel-haired ladies in musty, black coats and far fewer stooped men in ill-fitting suits would shuffle in and take their seats. Then, the music would start and the casket would be wheeled down the center aisle, shrouded with an embroidered cloth.

The mourners always seemed more tired than sad. From the moment the priest began with "*Requiem aeternam dona eis, Domine,*" the old people would take him at his word and begin dozing. "Grant them eternal rest, O Lord." They were often quite surprised to be wakened by our rendition of the Kyrie Eleison.

"We don't say the Requiem Mass anymore," Father Bob told me. "We try to make the commemorative service more a celebration of the person's life."

I craved the comfort of the ritual. I wanted Nick's body sent off with the familiar blessings. Father Bob agreed to do a regular mass, and we discussed the outlines of the service. I left him with checks for the organist, the soloist, and the printing of the program. There was no charge for the church, although I decided that later, after I was sure that my checks wouldn't bounce, I would send the church a modest donation.

In the four days since Nick's death, I have made arrangements for an evening memorial service, a morning funeral Mass, and a burial service, plus a catered reception to follow back at our house. Friends show up at all hours of the day and night, offering their help and bringing food and flowers. I am grateful for every one. There is a constant cycle of people sitting in the kitchen, drinking endless pots of coffee and tea to help ward off the chill. I offer beer, wine, and the limited selection of hard liquor that we have on hand, but no one seems in the mood for alcohol. My days have been crammed full of details—travel and hotel arrangements for out-of-town relatives, getting the kids outfitted, contacting florists and caterers. Yet, still time crawls. "You are holding everything together so well," everyone says. But inside, I feel like I'm torn apart.

We Are All
in It Together

Nick's mother sits beside me in the front pew, patting her eyes with a tissue, a small, white flag of surrender to her grief. Nikolaus offers to bring Matthew to the bathroom before the Mass begins. Over the past few days, Nikolaus has made a point of sticking with Matthew, keeping him busy and tending to his needs. I'm thankful for his help.

People begin to trickle in behind us, but no one comes up to the front where Elisabeth and I sit and wait. The air hums with muffled footsteps and murmured voices; the smell of damp wool mixes with candle wax and flowers. When I turn around to look for the boys, I am surprised to see how many people have come. Almost all of the seats are filled.

Nick and I were married in this church, but our wedding drew a much smaller crowd. There are no bride and groom sides now. Today, my sisters sit next to Nick's cousins. Today, we are all in it together.

I see lots of people I recognize, and many I don't. I know that some people have come a long way. I wonder if I should go around and greet everyone, thank them for coming. What would Jackie do? I decide to stay in my seat.

I see the Miners—the family of Nick's first wife, Rachael—sitting toward the back of the church. Nikolaus's grandparents, Ruth and LeRoy Miner, sit side by side. Their son, Rob Miner, sits next to his father. Rachael's younger sister, Nikolaus's Aunt Robyn, sits next to her mother. Rob catches my eye and gives me a faint nod. Rob has always been friendly and welcoming toward me. Ruth and Robyn, on the other hand, go out of their way to make me feel uncomfortable. I try not to take it personally. They wouldn't have liked anyone who came into Nick's life after Rachael. Robyn has never gotten over her sister's death. She doesn't want to. She honors her sister's memory mostly by being as openly hostile to me as she can. Although the seats next to Robyn are empty, Robyn's husband and two sons sit behind her, either by choice or because Robyn told them where to sit. This is not unusual. Although she's been married for over twenty years, Robyn's role as a daughter has always been more significant to her than her role as wife or mother.

The organist starts to play. The priest steps to the altar. Everyone stands, and the church doors open. Six men—Tom, my brother, and some of Nick's friends and coworkers—carry in the casket. Fat beads of rain quiver on the polished wood. The voice of a soloist fills the aisles, embracing the mourners, flooding all with warmth.

As the soloist's final note fades, Father Bob raises his arms and intones the opening prayers. Father Bob has known Nick for longer than I have. He said the Mass at Rachael's funeral; he married me and Nick. He dips his hand into a crystal bowl of holy water and sweeps the droplets over the casket in the sign of the cross. He indicates that the boys and I should do the same, each of us dribbling the blessed water over the polished surface, first one way and then the other. There is absolute silence in the crowded church as the ancient, time-honored ritual of the Mass begins.

As the boys and I return to our seats, Father Bob drapes the casket with an elaborately embroidered cloth. He balances a gold-leafed Bible on top of the draped surface and lets the book fall open to a page that has been marked with a crimson satin ribbon. He stands before the casket, arms raised, reciting the opening prayers in chanting tones, while shafts of light waft down from the clerestory windows, illuminating the gold-leafed pages from which he reads.

I am surprised at how familiar and comforting the prayers of the Mass are to me today, like hearing a favorite nursery poem told again after many years. Father Bob likes theatrical flourishes, which are keeping even the non-Christians entertained. He punctuates the rites with burning incense, chanting, and organ highlights that keep his audience spellbound. Near the end of the Mass, when he invites the congregation to come to the altar for either communion or a blessing, nearly everyone rises and moves forward.

After everyone is seated again, the religious ceremony is over and the personal part of the service begins. Matthew sits on my lap; Nikolaus sits next to me, holding my hand. I've asked four people to speak, each representing a different aspect of Nick's life. Nick's cousin Tom is first. He recalls how he and Nick grew up together in a rough East Oakland neighborhood. When Nick and his parents arrived in America, they lived, together with Tom's family, with an elderly uncle who had sponsored both families' entries into the United States. Tom and his parents and siblings eventually moved across the street to ease crowding at the uncle's house. Both Tom's and Nick's parents learned English from TV and an occasional night school class. Their fathers worked in factories or as delivery drivers—jobs with long hours of hard work that didn't require formal education or language skills. Their mothers cleaned houses and took in sewing, taking turns watching the children between jobs. Tom told the story of how Nick's father saved to buy a small plot of land in the Oakland hills and how the two families worked together to build a house on it. As teenagers, Nick, Tom, and Frank, Tom's brother, spent most nights and nearly every weekend pouring cement, hauling brick, putting up drywall, spackling, and painting.

They were fiercely loyal to each other, and Nick, as the oldest, watched out for the other kids. Nick put himself through college at UC Berkeley. He later earned an MBA in finance from the Golden Gate University—quite an accomplishment, considering that his mother left school before she learned to read. Nick and Tom had been best friends, closer than brothers. Losing Nick was even harder for Tom because his own brother had died unexpectedly five years ago after a brief illness. "It's hard to believe he's gone," Tom says, choking back tears. "It's hard to imagine a world without him."

Tom returns to his seat and Nick's friend Glenn replaces him at the podium. Nick and Glenn worked together for a number of years at Levi Strauss. They remained good friends throughout the years, despite Glenn's several job-related moves across the country.

Glenn remembers training with Nick for the San Francisco marathon. The two men prepared for months, rising at 5:00 AM for early-morning training, working out at lunchtime on San Francisco's steepest streets, and meeting on weekends for ten-mile runs. On the actual day of the race as they were nearing the finish line, Glenn got a debilitating leg cramp. "Nick refused to leave me," Glenn remembers. "He said that we trained together, and we were going to finish together. He held me up for the last mile of the race. I couldn't have done it without him."

Matthew is so quiet on my lap that I think he may have fallen asleep. But I see that his eyes are wide open and he is taking it all in, listening intently. How much of this will he remember? How much do I want him to remember?

Glenn is replaced at the podium by Steve, a colleague of Nick's from his current job at Mervyn's. Steve talks about Nick's care and concern for the people who worked with him and the people who worked for him. For a few years, Nick was the manager of a distribution center staffed mostly by hourly workers—hardworking people with minimal formal education and many recent immigrants with limited English. Steve talks about how Nick treated each of them with careful respect, recognized their contributions, and took pride in forming them into a successful team.

Steve closes with a story that illustrates Nick's love of contingency planning. One time he invited a team of managers to accompany him on a sailing trip on San Francisco Bay. "Nick was an experienced sailor, but few of us had ever sailed before," Steve recalls. "Nick greeted us at dockside with a sheet of typed instructions on what to do if he fell overboard, a possibility none of us had previously considered."

The story is so typical of Nick that even I have to smile. Nick liked to be prepared for any eventuality. Nick of course hadn't planned to die, but somehow I know he was ready in case the unthinkable did happen. I know that there are insurance policies. I know that he kept spreadsheets that I will be able to use to figure out our finances. But that is for another day. Today I have to figure out how to say goodbye.

The final speaker is LeRoy Miner. I brace myself, not sure what to expect. But LeRoy has always been careful not to take sides in the contentious relationship between his wife and me. He is, above all, a gentleman. He begins by saying that Nick was his son-in-law but also his friend. He says how thankful he was to Nick for taking care of his daughter in her last years, and that he knows how difficult those years were. He says how glad he was that Nick had been able to find someone else to build a life with after his daughter's death. He closes by thanking me for being a good mother to Nikolaus. "I'm proud that you are a part of our family."

The church is silent as he walks back to his seat. I can almost feel Ruth's eyes boring into my back. I dare not look back at her.

The organist strikes a sustained chord and then begins the recessional march. We walk slowly out of the church behind the casket, Elisabeth on Nikolaus's arm and me holding Matthew's hand. The sky is a thin blue. Dark, gray clouds hover at the edge of the horizon as we stand on the church steps and watch the casket disappear into the first of a series four black cars.

The stretch limo that brought us here is behind the hearse. Behind it are the other two limos, which I have not seen until now. One appears to be a relatively normal black town car, but I cringe when I see the other—a gleaming, black Rolls Royce with extravagantly curved bumpers and fat, white tires. Its front license plate reads, "Godfather Limos—Killer Style and Service." And there is not a thing I can do about it now.

The driver of the stretch limo holds the door open for us, and Elisabeth, the boys, and I step inside. The kids immediately begin fiddling with the TV. It pulls in only three channels—two snowy and one in Spanish. "I wish they had cable," Matthew complains. I pass the bag of granola bars and fruit I have brought along. Nikolaus takes two sodas from the bar and pours them into the highball glasses arranged on the TV cabinet.

Behind the darkened windows, I watch the people coming out onto the steps of the church. My family. The Miners. People I know. Neighbors, friends, clients, relatives. People I don't know. Nick's coworkers, childhood friends, neighbors. A whole lifetime's worth of people are huddled in small groups on the church steps.

My sister Jane knocks on the window. "Are you in there?" she asks, peering through the black glass. "Is there room for me?"

I open the door, and it takes her more than a few minutes to climb in. Jane's pregnant belly is huge. "I'm sorry to bother you, but I'm starved," she says. "I knew you'd bring snacks for the kids."

"Help yourself," Elisabeth says and passes her a granola bar. "You have to watch out for your baby."

"Who is the woman in the hat?" Jane asks. She points to a tall blond in a short, black dress who is picking her way down the church steps in three-inch heels, one hand steadying an enormous black hat.

"I think she works with Nick," I say.

"Elisabeth, you are holding up so well," Jane says, hugging her as best she can given the combination of sunken seating and Jane's huge stomach.

Elisabeth has, in fact, made it through the last few days with remarkable composure. I had feared the part of Elisabeth that is still of the Old World—the part that might wail over her son's body or throw herself down on the floor sobbing, dragging us all down with her. I feared these outbursts because I knew they would scare the children, who have remained so stoic, so composed, so numb. Just as I have. *Just wait until later,* I keep thinking. *Just let us get through the funeral. Then we can all have a good cry.*

Almost twenty minutes pass before the limos begin to pull away from the church with a trail of cars behind us. Time doesn't matter to me today. I have infinite patience. Our car follows the hearse down the streets of the town that Nick lived in for most of his life. We pass streets full of people in the middle of their normal everyday existence—carrying groceries or dry cleaning, standing in line for coffee or lunch, waiting for the bus. I see some turn to watch the hearse drive by, followed by the three ill-matched black limos and then the long line of cars. Do they wonder if it's someone they know in that hearse? Do they think about the fact that someday it will be them? We don't come close to the parade Jackie organized, but in this small town, I still feel like we are putting on a show.

We turn toward the highway, passing car dealerships and fast food chains.

"Can we pull into one of these places for a minute so I can go to the bathroom?" my sister asks. "I'm sorry, but this baby is pressing on my bladder."

"There are at fifty cars following us, Ma'am," the driver says. "If we pull into a burger place, they will, too."

We drive through the wide, iron gates of the cemetery and wind our way past the rows of stone—first the large, elaborate ones dating from the early 1900s, then the smaller, more recent slabs adorned with plastic flowers.

On television, mourners always stand at the side of the grave. "It's quite expensive to have a graveside service," the funeral director had told me, ever mindful of my budget. "We'd have to rent a canopy and chairs. And at this time of year, they will require that we lay artificial turf over the adjacent graves."

"So we won't get muddy?" I asked.

"Actually, it's done to preserve the lawn," he said. "Believe me, everyone's shoes will still get muddy. That's something you might want to think about if you are planning to invite people back to your house afterward." I pictured cemetery dirt tracked over the kitchen floor and ground into the carpet. I pictured fifty pairs of muddy shoes lined up next to my front door and everyone standing around in bare feet. I bet Jackie didn't have to worry about mourners tracking mud through the White House.

"Let's stick with the chapel then," I decided.

So now we head toward the chapel for final interment prayers. Then we will leave Nick here and go back home. Tonight, when all the mourners are gone, cemetery workers will use a crane to lower him into the earth and a backhoe to cover him with fresh dirt. This is what happens in real life.

Carved limestone saints look down at us as we climb the stairs to the heavy, gilded doors of the main chapel. Jane makes a beeline to the bathroom. The rest of us quickly fill the two-dozen rows of carved wooden benches. Nick's casket is carried in and placed in the center aisle, covered with a spray of red roses.

"Are we not going to the grave?" Elisabeth whispers.

"No," I whisper back. "We have to say goodbye here."

"Oh." She does not look happy.

I feel bad about adding to her sorrow on this day but there is nothing I can do. The plans are set.

The final blessings echo against the marble walls. Father Bob chants, "Eternal rest grant unto him, O Lord. And let perpetual light shine upon him," and we answer, "May he rest in peace. Amen." It is all over very quickly.

"I want to see him in the grave," Elisabeth insists as we begin to file out of the small chapel.

"It's just not the way things work here," I say. I know that this is not a sufficient explanation, but what else can I say to her?

Father Bob asks if I want to take a rose from the casket spray. I shake my head. I don't want anything that will remind me of this day. I run my hand lightly over the gleaming brass trim. Nikolaus raises his hand in a small sign of farewell. Matthew pulls a rose off and tucks it in his pocket. His hand leaves a trail of tiny fingerprints on the glossy wood. I hold Matthew's hand as we walk down the center aisle. We have almost reached the doorway when I hear someone sobbing. At the same moment, I realize

Elisabeth is no longer behind me. I turn around and see that she has thrown herself across the casket and is sobbing loudly.

"Oh, Nicky, Nicky," she moans. "Why did you have to go? You are so young still!"

I tell Matthew to wait for me on the steps and rush to her side. Nikolaus tries to lift Elisabeth by the arm, but she resists. It takes both of us to pry her away from the casket and drag her, sobbing, out the door.

The outside air calms her a bit, and we pause for a moment to help her catch her breath before descending the steep steps. Looking out over the soggy lawn, I can see Nick's grave marked by a huge pile of freshly dug earth and a mound of flowers delivered from the funeral home.

"Why can't we wait while they put him in the grave?" Elisabeth moans.

"He'll stay in the chapel until after the cemetery closes," I answer. "They use big machines to fill the grave. They told me that they can't bury him while people are here."

A memory comes to me, suddenly, unbidden. I was in high school. A good friend of mine had committed suicide, and after the funeral service, I climbed up through the weeds on the hill overlooking the small cemetery at the edge of town. I waited and watched until, about an hour later, the crane came. The crane operator stooped to place bright orange straps around the shiny white box. Then, in a moment, the casket was hoisted high in the air. I held my breath as it twisted and swung on its fragile tether. For several minutes, it seemed adrift against the bright blue sky. Then the crane skillfully fit the small, white box into the open hole below. That was my friend's last moment in the sun, and I was there. The thump as the casket hit bottom took a few seconds to echo up the hill. I watched the backhoe scoop a great mound of dirt back into the open hole, then press it down until it was level. When it was done and I was sure that all the workers had left, I climbed down to lay wildflowers I had gathered—weeds, in truth—on the dark brown rectangle.

"How do we know they will bury him?" Elisabeth asks.

"They'll take good care of him," I say. "He's with God now." I put my arm around her as I help her down the stairs. "We have to go now. People will be coming to the house soon."

Nikolaus and Matthew have already climbed inside the limo and are playing with the TV again. Just as I'm about to climb in, I see Ruth Miner walking toward us. "Our family is not going to the house," she says.

"I'm so sorry you can't make it," I say graciously. *Jackie would be proud of me,* I think, and assuming that that's the end of the conversation, I turn to get into the car. But behind me, Ruth continues. "I will call you in a few days to talk about what will happen to Nikolaus now," she says.

I don't understand what she means, but when I turn back to ask her, she is already walking away.

One Great Party

chapter five

By the time we get back to the house, it is raining again. The three limos follow each other up the long driveway to our house. The drivers' doors open with perfect precision. Three large, black umbrellas mushroom out and form a slow procession up the front stairs, with the three drivers escorting Elisabeth, my mother, and my sister. My brother, John, and his wife trail behind them, while Nikolaus and Matthew try to beat each other in a run for the open front door. They are running and laughing and falling over each other like puppies. I'm amazed at their ability to find joy on this awful day, if only for a moment, and grateful for their resilience.

My friend Karin is waiting inside the house. A few years ago, I was hired by the vice president of a big company to write a marketing plan for a new product. Karin was the product manager. We got along great. She eventually got a job with a different company and hired me to write some brochures. Although we've been working closely together and been friends for three or four years, I don't think she'd ever been to my house. Three days after Nick died, she showed up on my doorstep. "I heard," she said simply. "What can I do to help?" She offered to stay in the house during the funeral and fend off the burglars that supposedly prowl the homes of grieving families attending memorial services. Scanning the obituary page for burglary targets seems like a specious strategy to me, but my mother insisted that it happens all the time. I needed someone to let the caterers in anyway, and Karin was willing. Although she and I had worked together for several years, she had only met Nick once or twice. "I don't mind missing the funeral," she assured me. "I don't do organized religion well."

I sit in the car, alone for a moment, reluctant to leave the quiet, gray leather cocoon. Behind the darkened windows, I see my Uncle Babe standing on the front porch. As each driver turns away from the door, he gives each one a solemn and slightly prolonged handshake. It takes me a minute to realize that he is slipping each one a tip.

I come up behind him as the last driver walks back toward the limos. "You didn't have to do that," I whisper. "I'm already paying a fortune for those cars."

He smiles and pats my hand. "They have families to feed."

My uncle is called Babe because he is youngest of three brothers; my father, who has been dead five years now, was the oldest. The family still calls him Babe, even though he stands over six feet tall and is almost eighty years old. The family has always called the three brothers—my father, Babe, and Vincent—"the boys," although they haven't been boys for decades. My sisters, brother, and I will forever be "the kids," even as we move into our forties. My family is accustomed to longevity, and things change very slowly, if at all.

"I'm so sorry that you and Uncle Vincent had to ride in the Godfather car."

He raises his eyebrows in mock surprise. "What's to be sorry about? After all, Uncle Vincent is your godfather, isn't he?" His eyes sparkle with mischief. "He thinks you ordered that car especially for him. Better not to tell him if you didn't."

I follow my uncle inside. Karin and the caterers have worked magic while we were at the service—I can't remember the house ever looking so good. Nick would have been so pleased; he loved it when the house was spiffed up and ready for guests. The dozens of floral displays that have been delivered to us over the past few days are arranged throughout the rooms like small sparks of life. Larger displays decorate the living room mantel and the table in the hall. The dining room table showcases an array of meats and salads and breads, and there is a bar set up in the family room. Everything looks great, but neither the food nor the drink appeals to me.

My mother and sisters bustle around doing things that probably don't need to be done. Elisabeth and the uncles hover over the boys, making them change into dry shoes and getting them to eat before the crowd comes. I figure it is best just to stay out of the way. I sit in the living room, breathing in the gentle fragrance of the flowers. Through the sliding glass doors, I see dark clouds moving slowly across the distant horizon. Nick's face smiles out from a frame over the fireplace. Someone suggested that I take a picture of Nick, blow it up, and place it next to the casket at the memorial service. That way people would remember what he looked like in life rather than what he looked like in the casket. In the photo, Nick's dark hair tumbles across his forehead and his eyes are warm and sparkling.

Elisabeth insisted on leaving the casket open during the memorial service. Laid out on ripples of white satin, Nick looked like hell, but then, who wouldn't with eyes and mouth sewn shut? I was horrified when I saw him. Jackie had refused to let her husband be seen that way, but Elisabeth wouldn't hear of closing the lid. "This is the last time I'll ever see him," she said, sadly. She asked one of her friends to take pictures of Nick to send to relatives back in Germany. I wish that Elisabeth and the boys could have seen him on the day he died, the way he looked in the hospital—slightly disheveled, cold and still, but perfect.

Smaller photos of Nick surround the large one on the mantel and spill over onto tables scattered around the room. Over the past few days, Tina and I sorted through boxes of photos, most still enclosed in drugstore envelopes, looking for pictures of Nick. Through the years, Nick and I had taken very few pictures of each other; most of our pictures were of the kids. After sifting through hundreds of photos, we were only able to find two dozen or so that showed Nick, and even in those he was mostly in a supporting role—shaving Matthew's hair into a buzz cut, steadying Nikolaus's first two-wheeled bike, standing behind a line of Cub Scouts proudly displaying their pinewood derby cars. Tom had brought over some of Nick's childhood pictures, and we spent an afternoon putting all the pictures into inexpensive frames we had bought in bulk quantities.

"What is this doing here?" I hear Jane ask from behind me, pointing to the photo of Nick's first wedding. Nick's and Rachael's families are fanned out on both sides of the couple. Both mothers sport stiff beehive hairdos. Jane examines the photo for a minute and then says, "It's really an odd wedding picture. Nobody looks very happy."

"They weren't happy. Nick's family was totally against the marriage because Rachael was sick and needed constant care. And the Miners—well, Ruth Miner, anyway—didn't think that Nick was capable of taking care of her."

"It was nice of LeRoy Miner to acknowledge your part in

raising Nikolaus, even though Nick had to die before he did it."
Jane is always on my side. I love her for that.

I have been waiting for a moment alone with Jane to ask her
a big favor. As we stand there reviewing the pictures, I summon
up the energy to discuss the problem of Nick's will.

Nick had a will, of course. There is no way Nick would neglect something so important. He was very careful about things
like that. For Nick, death was not an abstract concept—it was
a reality, and he knew the consequences. He had been through
Rachael's death and then, shortly after, his own father's. When I
first met him, he was still trying to finalize both their estates.

Just before we got married, Nick and I picked a lawyer out of
the phone book and made an appointment to update our wills. At
the same time, we had a short prenuptial agreement drawn. After
all, we were not rosy-cheeked children when we got married. We
were both over thirty. We had careers—he in management, I in
marketing. We had investments. We had plans.

And there was Nikolaus to consider. "If something happens
to me, I want Nikolaus to grow up in a family," Nick said. This
made sense to me. I had only known Nick and Nikolaus for a
little over a year. Getting married was a huge step for me. Taking
responsibility for a six-year-old child was even bigger.

We asked the lawyer if I should formally adopt Nikolaus.
"There's no real need," he advised us. "As long as you are married to the child's natural father, you are, in effect, his mother.
Formally adopting him is a nice thing to do, but it's expensive
and unnecessary."

Nick decided to name Rob Miner, Rachael's brother, as Nikolaus's guardian should something happen to Nick. Rob and his
wife were still together then, and they had three children, nice
kids, the youngest only a year older than Nikolaus. At the time, it
seemed like the right thing to do—the best thing for Nikolaus in
case the worst happened.

By the time Matthew was born, four years later, a lot had changed. Our marriage was strong, our assets commingled, and I had become Nikolaus's mother. I'd been helping Nikolaus with his homework, listening to his piano lessons, managing his Scouts projects, chaperoning his class trips. I was his mother, no matter what my legal standing. I knew his routines, his likes and dislikes, his friends. Since Nick and I had to update our wills to include Matthew, it now made sense to also change Nikolaus's guardianship from Rob Miner to me.

Through work, Nick was enrolled in a ten-dollar-a-month, 1-800-number legal service. Within a week of calling, we received a package of forms. It took us several weeks, as we had other priorities, like feeding and changing baby Matthew, to complete and return them. The forms required us to make decisions about who would get our worldly assets (we named each other), who would become guardian for the children (we named each other), and who would be executor and trustee of our estates (we named each other). What we got back by return mail were standard legal wills that would have trumped all the prenuptial agreements, guardianships, and other divisions that convoluted the previous paperwork. They only needed to be signed by us and two disinterested witnesses.

And herein lay our fundamental oversight, or laziness. Nick and I would have signed them immediately but for the requirement that our signatures be witnessed by two disinterested parties. Any of our friends could have been witnesses. But there never seemed to be a right time to ask them. "Come to dinner tonight, and would you mind being witnesses for our wills over dessert?" On the day Nick died, our wills sat in a folder on the desk in the kitchen, still unsigned, still unwitnessed.

So, one of my major concerns in the days following Nick's death was whether or not I had any legal right to remain as Nikolaus's mother, or if Rob Miner now automatically would become his legal guardian. I wasn't sure. Regardless of who Nikolaus's legal guardian was, certainly it made more sense for him to stay with me and with Matthew; we were his family. Surely Rob would see that. I was Nikolaus's best hope for maintaining his current life—and he was mine. I didn't want to let him down. But the Miners were Nikolaus's blood relatives, a fact they never let me forget. I was not blood. And I was not the guardian named in his father's only valid will.

Since the day that Nick died, I have been trying to work up the nerve to forge his signature on the new will, the one that would make me Nikolaus's guardian. Then I could fake the witness signatures, I figure, and that would be that. I just haven't been able to work up the necessary mindset for all this forging and faking. My other alternative is to forge Nick's signature and then ask someone else to "witness" it. This means asking someone to lie for me, to pretend they signed the papers before Nick died. I know that Jane would understand my predicament, and I know that she would do it if I asked her to. Maybe she would even help me forge another signature for the second witness. And so I have just been waiting—postponing—for the right time to ask her.

"You girls come and eat something now," my mother calls to us from the dining room. "People will be coming very soon."

In fact, people are already arriving. I decide to wait to talk to Jane about the will. I hear the babble of greetings from the front hall. It is still raining. It was a lousy day for a funeral.

My mother fills a plate with chicken salad, a buttered roll, mixed fruit, and a deviled egg and hands it to me. I take a bite of the chicken salad. It is as tasteless as water and feels unpleasantly lumpy in my mouth. When I swallow, it sticks in my throat. "Isn't that chicken salad delicious?" my mother asks. I nod. Satisfied, she goes off to greet someone in the next room. I stand where I am, holding the plate firmly and looking down at the food that I know is impossible for me to eat.

People are wandering into the dining room, no doubt encouraged by my mother. They murmur a soft litany. "So sorry," the voices say. "Such a shock." "I just can't believe it." They want to hug me, but I'm holding the plate of food so there is an awkward moment before they pat my back or squeeze my arm instead. I try to think about what Jackie would say to smooth their discomfiture, to recognize their good intentions. "Thank you so much for coming," I say. "It's wonderful to know that so many people care about us."

The dining room is drawing a crowd. Everyone but me is hungry. I carry my plate back into the living room, looking for escape, but the living room is crowded now, too. A woman I don't recognize murmurs her sympathy. "Can I get you something to drink?" she asks. She is wearing a black sweater and slacks. I try to place her. She looks at me expectantly, kindly.

I shake my head. "Thank you so much for coming," I tell her. "It's wonderful to know that so many people care about us."

"I'm Lucy," she replies. "I'm with the catering company."

I see my mother working her way across the room toward me. I don't want her to see the untouched plate of food. "Lucy, can you please get rid of this plate for me?"

My mother is getting closer, but I pretend not to notice her until Lucy and the plate are safely out of sight.

"Don't worry," my mother says in a low voice as she reaches my side and grabs my arm, "I've explained to everyone why you are wearing red."

"What a relief," I say. "I'm going to get a drink."

A table in the family room holds a display of glassware and several types of wine, beer, and soda. Someone hands me a glass of wine. I take a sip. It tastes sour and burns along the edges of my throat. Karin is standing next to me. "Is the wine okay?" I ask her. "It tastes bad to me."

"It's very good, actually," she says.

"It must just be me then."

"I bet there's a hundred people here." Karin is practically shouting in my ear, but she has to speak loudly to be heard above the babble of conversation around us.

It is, by far, the largest gathering we have ever had. Everyone seems to be having a good time. I can't help but think about Nick not being here to enjoy it. He loved having people over, loved being the host. As I move from room to room through the crowd, I expect to hear his voice, his laugh.

My friend Janine sidles up next to me. "I feel like Nick is here with us," she says.

"Do you really?" I ask, surprised.

Karin shakes her head. "I don't think it's possible for his spirit to be among us today." Karin is skeptical of mainstream religions, but she is an enthusiastic proponent of ancient beliefs, talismans, and rites. "Buddha teaches that the spirit can only stay around for three days before it has to move on to another life."

"I thought it was three weeks," Janine says.

Karin is serene but firm. "No, it's definitely three days."

Someone else chimes in. "Is it three days from the date of death, or three days from the date of burial?"

I say, "I think I'll go get some air," but I don't think anyone hears me.

Outside, the rain has stopped, and the air is cool and fresh. I close the sliding door behind me and cross the deck to the steps that lead up behind the house, out of sight to those inside. At the top of the steps is a familiar figure, bathed in halo of smoke. "Annemarie, is that you?" I ask, recognizing my friend and neighbor. "Are you smoking?"

She gives me a guilty grin. "Just needed one," she says. "I don't want the kids to see me." Annemarie has a daughter, Leigh, who is in high school with Nikolaus.

"When did you start smoking?" I ask.

"Oh, I don't really smoke," she says, exhaling a long, thick stream. "I just do it when I'm upset. It calms me down."

We stand in silence for a moment, and then she says, "I filed divorce papers yesterday."

I'm really surprised. I have known Annemarie and her husband, Kurt, since we moved to this neighborhood ten years ago. We first met when we served together on some long-forgotten school committee, and our friendship grew from there. "What happened?" I ask, although I think I already know.

"Nothing happened," she says, taking another long drag and then letting it slowly out. "Nothing is ever going to happen. He's wrapped up in his business, in his motorcycle, and in whatever sport is in season at the moment. He's not wrapped up in what's happening with Leigh or with me." She shrugs, drops the cigarette butt on the concrete, and grinds it out with her heel.

"I'm sorry." I don't know what else to say.

"Yeah, I'm sorry, too." Annemarie pulls another cigarette out of a half-empty pack and tamps the end against her palm, the practiced move of a habitual smoker. "But I'll be damned if I'm going to live the rest of my life trying to get someone's attention. So, I decided to end it. Life's too short, I just want to go for it."

I don't ask her what she is going for. I know she doesn't know.

"I'm sorry to burden you with all of this," she says. "Especially today. You have enough trouble of your own."

"Actually, this is the first conversation I've had all week where I actually forgot my troubles for a moment." I am surprised at how normal I suddenly feel.

Annemarie laughs. "Well, see? Good things are coming from this divorce already." She gazes down at the unlit cigarette still in her hand, then shrugs and carefully inserts it back into the pack. "Look, I have to be going. I'm not much good around people today."

"How about if I call you tomorrow?"

"You have your hands full with family and all right now. I'll wait until everyone's gone, and then I'll call you."

"Deal," I agree. "Now I better get back inside."

A Clear
Message

People continue to come and go throughout the afternoon and well into the evening hours. Jane takes a cab back to the hotel around five o'clock; it had been a long day for her and the baby. My brother and his wife left earlier; they have an early morning flight. By eight, the caterers are cleaning up and Elisabeth, my mother, my sister Judy, Karin, and I are sitting around the kitchen table, drinking tea.

"It's a good thing we hired the caterers," Judy says. "You'll have leftovers to eat all next week."

"Did you have enough to eat?" my mother asks me.

"Yes, Mom," I lie.

"You don't have to worry about meals for the next month," Karin says. "While you were at the services this morning, people kept dropping by with flowers and pans of food. I put it all in your freezer in the garage. Lasagna seems to be the dish of choice. You have enough to feed an army."

Lucy, the caterer, comes in from the front hall and says, "I'm sorry to bother you, but I can't find the switch for the front-porch lights. Can you help?"

I get up and follow her back into the hall. "It's this one right here by the door." I flick the switch but nothing happens.

"Maybe the bulb is burned out," Lucy suggests.

"It might be," I say, "but there are three bulbs in that fixture. They don't usually all go out at once." I flick the switch a few more times. "Maybe the switch is bad."

"It's really dark out there," Lucy says.

"How about if you go out the back way?" I suggest. "It's a few steps longer, but at least there'll be some light."

"What's wrong?" my mother calls from the kitchen.

"Nothing, Mom. Just some burned-out lights." I head over to the back door and flip that light switch on. Peering out the door, I see that it's still pitch black. I flip the switch back down and then up again firmly. Nothing.

"What's going on?" Karin asks.

"None of the outside lights seem to be working," I explain.

"Maybe it's a short circuit," Judy suggests. "Want me to go look at the circuit box?"

"No," I say quickly. The front and back porch lights are on different circuits; if either circuit was blown, the lights in the living room and kitchen would be off, too, not just the outside lights. "I'll just get a lantern."

"I wish Nicky were here," Elisabeth says. "He could fix anything."

"He had golden hands," my mother agrees.

"But Nicky is not here," Elisabeth says, her eyes pooling up.

"Maybe Nick is here," Karin says quietly. "Maybe the lights are his message to us."

Elisabeth looks up from her tissue. "There are no messages," she says. "When you are dead, that's it. You are dead."

A Clear Message

"There have been documented instances of the dead sending messages through electrical circuits," Karin insists.

"What do you think Nick is trying to say?" Judy asks her. I can't tell if she is genuinely interested or just humoring Karin. Either way, the conversation is getting on my nerves.

"I think he's saying that it's time to get some lanterns," I interrupt, and I grab a flashlight and head out to the garage. The dark doesn't scare me, and I feel Nick's absence much more keenly than I feel his presence. If Nick were here, I would want him to be fixing the lights, not breaking them. Nick knows that I'm not good at dealing with electrical problems. Karin is right about one thing, though. The sudden lack of lights is sending me a very clear message: I'm in the dark, and I'm on my own. And that thought is scarier to me than any ghost story could ever be.

Always and Forever

chapter seven

The morning after the funeral, Elisabeth, the kids, and I meet my family for breakfast at their hotel. Everyone is leaving today, going back to their own homes and their own lives.

"Tomorrow, everything will be back to normal," my mother sighs over her French toast. Jane elbows her sharply. I pretend not to notice.

I'm distracted anyway. I haven't been able to ask my sisters to help me sign Nick's will—I just couldn't find the ideal moment to ask them to forge a legal document. Now, it's too late. I'll have to ask Karin or Janine to do it. Or I'll just make up names and fake the signatures. I'll decide what to do later.

After breakfast, I send Nikolaus upstairs to help coordinate and carry the luggage, and Matthew insists on tagging along to help. My mother and Elisabeth retreat to my mother's room to call the various airlines to make sure that everyone's flights are on schedule. My mother and Elisabeth enjoy each other's company, and they like to be helpful, even though they spend more time chatting than phoning.

Although it had been raining earlier, now the sky looks mercifully clear. My uncles find me sitting in the lobby and invite me to go with them for a short walk. We head for the hotel's garden.

"It's hard to believe that it's February," Uncle Vincent says, stopping to admire a row of flowers. "Back in New York, it's twenty degrees and snowing. Here, daffodils are blooming."

"So, you are thinking of moving out here?" I pretend it's a serious question.

He chuckles. "You know the answer to that." My uncles have spent eighty years in New York and are probably never going to leave. "But I hope you also know that you can always come 'back east,' as they say out here."

"I'm not sure what I'll do now," I say. Uncle Babe walks just slightly ahead of us. He is listening, but he always lets Vincent handle the heavy discussions. He calls Vincent "The Communicator" in a teasing way that still conveys his respect for his older brother.

"If we moved back east," I continue, "I'd be nearer my family, but it would be very disruptive for the kids. They've never lived anywhere but here."

"Family will help you wherever you are. Friends will only help you if they are close. But judging by the crowd at the house yesterday and the amount of lasagna in your freezer, you have a lot of friends here. Let them help you. You'll need them now."

"I'll be fine," I assure him. "I have Elisabeth, too. She helps me."

"Nick's death will be hardest on Elisabeth." Vincent shakes his head sadly. "To lose a child, even a grown child, is a terrible tragedy."

"It will be difficult for her to cope without Nick," I say. "He took care of her house, handled her medicines, paid her bills. I'll have to do all of that now. I wonder if it wouldn't be easier if she just moved in with us."

We stop before a small, empty flowerbed. Uncle Babe is stooped down, using his finger to trace an outline in the fresh dirt. As we watch, he draws two stick figures side by side and then connects them with a heavy, straight line that rests on the top of their circle heads.

When he is done, he stands straight and rubs the dirt off his fingers thoughtfully. "What is it?" I ask.

"It's the Chinese symbol for unhappiness," Babe says slowly. "Two women under one roof."

—⁓—

It is Saturday, February 14. It is Valentine's Day. It's exactly one week since the day Nick died.

At 8:30 AM, the doorbell rings. When I open the door, a dozen long-stemmed red roses are thrust into my hands. "Happy Valentine's Day!" the man chirps. He is already at the bottom of the steps, speeding off to his next delivery. I know immediately who these flowers are from. My mother-in-law peers over the stairs.

"Who is it, Gloria?" she asks.

"Just more flowers," I say. Sympathy arrangements of lilies, statices, and white roses still crowd the living and family rooms. Potted azaleas, orchids, and dieffenbachia line the kitchen counters and front hall.

"Who can these be from?" Elisabeth asks.

"From my sisters," I lie. "For Valentine's Day."

Roses in hand, I retreat to my bedroom and close the door. I pull the tiny card out of the envelope and read the message I knew would be there. It had been there every year for the past ten years.

"I love you, always and forever. Nick."

Always and Forever

—⚇—

On Sunday, Elisabeth drags her big, black suitcase down the staircase into the living room. "I go home today," she announces. "You don't have to leave," I say. "You know you can stay as long as you want."

"I know this, honey," Elisabeth said. "And I thank you for this. But I think I go home."

"Did my uncles talk to you?" I ask, but Elisabeth doesn't seem to know what I am talking about.

Home Sweet Home

chapter eight

What I remember most about the days after the funeral is the rain. No soothing, gentle rain, but a relentless, unending stream pouring from a leaden sky that made large parts of the surrounding hills dissolve into great rivers of mud that swirled down into unlucky streets. Backyard pools pushed up out of the swollen soil, and homes groaned on shifting foundations. Still the rain continued to pound against the roof and windows, drowning all other sound or thought, draining life and color out of everything. The weather matched my mood. Inside, I felt drab and dead. The only clothes I felt comfortable in were in shades of black and gray. Color hurt my eyes.

In the calm places, when the rain subsided and the wind died down, I'd pull on rubber boots and climb up to take a closer look at the hillside behind our house. Nick was always watching the hill for the landslides that are common in our area. Last fall, in anticipation of heavy winter rains, Nick and I covered the top part of the hill with great sheets of black plastic to prevent it from washing away. I fuss with the plastic now, rearranging the edges under the heavy railroad ties that hold it down. I look for signs of erosion, for signs of danger. Actually, I'm not really sure what I am looking for or that I'll know what to do when I see it.

Over the ten years we've lived in this house, Nick and I have brought in more than thirty tons of rock, which lie in long, gray ribbons along the bottom of each slope. "Other men might buy their wives diamonds," Nick once joked, standing next to yet another truckload of rock, "but I get you truckloads of real rocks." I pick my way carefully over the jagged rock ribbons, watching the rainwater drain between them and thinking how stupidly special each one is to me now.

Climbing to the top of the hill, I can look down on the house and yard below. From here, it all looks small and easily managed. In fact, this house has been a stretch for us financially, physically, and time-wise ever since we bought it. "Our strategy," Nick said when we first talked about marriage, "will be to buy the worst house in the best neighborhood that we can afford. Then, we can fix it up."

This house was so important to him because it represented everything he had aspired to when he was a child living with relatives in a deteriorating neighborhood. Nick worked hard to give his kids the things he had never had: a backyard, safe streets, good schools.

We were able to buy this house because the price had been reduced several times as other buyers shied away from the amount of work it obviously needed. For the first five years, we lived with stained carpets, dingy wallpaper, sagging decks, and leaky windows. We spent all our free time building what Nick called "sweat equity": scraping the cottage cheese coating off the ceilings, laying fresh linoleum in the bathrooms, digging out the weeds that choked the garden.

It was a long time before we felt comfortable with our neighbors. They all seemed to have gardeners, cleaning services, and professional nannies. They escaped to their Tahoe cabins or planned exotic vacations while we struggled from paycheck to paycheck.

Now, ten years later, we had completed most of the remodeling and repairs. "We are down to routine maintenance now," Nick said last spring. The redwood trees we planted that first year now stand over thirty feet tall. Nick had paced off their planting holes eight feet apart, which seemed like an enormous distance then. Now their branches intertwine, producing small sprays of raindrops, like showers of tears, as I brush through them.

I stand at the top of the hill and look at all the dreams we had that have come true. If Nick were here today, I know that this is where I'd find him. I strain to hear his voice in the whisper of the grass, in the rustle of the trees. I hear nothing. I try to feel his presence in this place he loved more than any other. I feel only alone and small, daunted by everything that Nick dreamed and accomplished, overwhelmed by the relatively little that is left now for me to do.

PART 2 Planet Widow

Back to Normal

chapter nine

I thought that once the funeral was over, we would pick up the pieces of our life and simply go on. There would always be a void, of course, a place where Nick was supposed to be but wasn't. We would be sad for a while, but we would survive. The truth is, I wasn't at all prepared for how much my life was about to change.

It's Monday, time for the boys to be back in school. I stand on the front porch and watch Nikolaus walk down our long driveway. His step is light and springy; his backpack bobs happily on his back. He is glad to be rejoining the world. I don't want to let him go. When he is out of my sight, anything can happen.

Matthew is more reluctant to leave. "I could stay home and keep you company," he offers.

"Your teacher and friends at school are missing you," I answer, pulling his sweatshirt over his head.

He looks concerned. "Are you going to cry today?" He has seen me cry a few times over the past couple of days, and it has him worried. I want to show him that it's okay to cry, something he's been desperately avoiding. On the other hand, I don't want him worrying about me while he is in school.

"I won't cry today," I promise. "I have too many things to do."

I drop him off in front of his school and watch him trudge toward his classroom, the weight of his worry hunching his shoulders and dragging his steps.

Back home, there is a stack of unopened mail waiting. Every day, the mailbox has been stuffed full. Much of the mail is sympathy cards, which I have been separating from the bills and other mail. I can only open a few cards at a time. On many of them, people have taken the time to write a few words of comfort, an offer of help. The ones that include a memory of Nick–something they did together, something he said to them once–are my favorites. But I can't look at them today because I've promised Matthew I wouldn't cry.

Upstairs in my office, a stack of financial papers waits for my attention. It is a combination of tax records and receipts, insurance records, bills, and bank statements. Everything I need to know about our finances is probably in this pile. And there is a lot that I need to know.

Nick and I shared financial responsibilities, so I am not totally in the dark with regard to our finances. We put a portion of our paychecks into a joint checking account that we used to pay house bills. Nick usually wrote the checks, but I know exactly how much the mortgage payment is and about how much the monthly bills run. There was seldom money left over at the end of the month; in fact, we often ran short. We were barely making it on two paychecks. I know that we can't make it on my paycheck alone.

We do have other resources I can draw on–at least, in the short term. Every time Nick got a bonus check or I got a windfall from an extra project, we used the extra money to fund college savings accounts for each of the kids. We also put some money aside in a general investment account. While these accounts aren't large, they are accessible. But since Nikolaus will begin applying to colleges next year, I have to be careful about using that money. Depending on what college Nikolaus chooses, I will soon need Nikolaus's fund, and possibly some of the investment money, as well.

If I get desperate, my family would gladly help me out. But I'd have to be starving or one step away from living on the street before I'd ask them. It would be hard to justify asking my mother or my uncles to share their retirement nest eggs just so that we could maintain a big house or the kids could go to private colleges. The fact is, we will just have to scale back and learn to live within reduced means.

There are also retirement accounts that I can draw on if I really get into trouble. Nick was very serious about saving for retirement. He had the maximum deducted from his paycheck to fund a retirement account. "I don't want to work for the rest of my life," he often said. "There are so many things I want to do." I can't think of anything I want to do now, without him.

I know that if I were smart enough, I could develop a financial strategy that would help me get through. But I'm not that smart. Nick was very smart about money. Savings and investment strategies were a constant source of conflict between us. Nick thought I was too conservative, and I felt that he was way too aggressive. Nick came from an immigrant family, people who had bet everything on the chance for a better life. I was raised by parents who lived through the Depression, conservative people who valued security above all else. I distrust easy money; Nick believed in opportunity.

I'm not sure where our finances stand at this point, but I know that the answer lies in that pile of paper. I'm not anxious to dive in. I already know that I can't afford the mortgage on my paycheck. What I don't know is how long I have before they will foreclose. I know that we are still paying off the home-equity line we took out to remodel the house, but I don't know exactly what the balance is or how I will pay it. I don't know exactly what our credit card balances are, but I suspect that they're big. I know that Nick's company had a life insurance plan, but it has occurred to me that it may not pay off since he didn't die on the job. We had medical and dental insurance through Nick's company, and I'm not sure we'll still be eligible now.

I pull my desk chair over to the pile and pick up the top paper. It's a bank statement from our joint account. The balance is $6,000. This is good. I look at the statement date. It's from last November, before Christmas expenses. This is not good. I put the statement aside.

Next in the pile is a bill from one of Nick's credit cards. The balance due is just over $8,000. I want to look away, but I force myself to keep my eyes on the bottom line. I can't seem to catch my breath.

Don't panic, I tell myself. *Don't waste time feeling sorry for yourself.*

Then I start to think that going through what I owe is the wrong approach. Maybe the best thing to do is just to get back to work as soon as possible. I have two projects going—if I can finish them quickly, I can get paid. I decide to call one of my clients, Doug, and try to reschedule a meeting I had cancelled last week.

His secretary puts me through immediately.

"How are you?" Doug's voice oozes with sympathy. "I didn't expect to hear from you so soon."

"Well, I know I left you hanging last week on that presentation, so I thought I'd call. . . ."

"Oh my God, don't even think about the presentation," he says. "You have much more important things to take care of."

"I have the presentation done," I go on doggedly. "I thought we could reschedule. . . ."

"Everyone here understands what you're going through," he says. "We've agreed to put the project on hold until things have settled down for you."

"Well, thanks, but . . ."

"Just take whatever time you need now to get yourself and your kids settled. Don't worry about the project. It'll wait for you. I'll call you in a few weeks."

He hangs up. I am left holding the phone, wondering what to do next. I briefly consider calling him back but decide against it. I don't want to appear too desperate.

I am also working on a project for the investment firm, Charles Schwab. Schwab was one of my first clients; I've worked for the company on and off for more than six years doing marketing plans and writing investor education programs on topics such as saving for retirement and investing for your child's education. In fact, I've been at Schwab so long that many people are surprised when they learn I'm not a regular employee.

On this particular project, developing a plan for a mail advertising campaign, I'm working with a group of people I really enjoy. I can level with them if I have to. I can beg if I need to. I should have called them first.

Melanie is my main contact for this project. She is not in when I call. "Call me as soon as you can," I say to her voice mail.

I'm feeling weak and lightheaded. I realize this is probably because I haven't eaten yet today. I've always been more likely to drown my sorrows in a hot fudge sundae than in booze. But now, I seem to have lost interest in both food and drink. Chewing seems like a huge effort, my throat too tight to swallow. And anything I do manage to get down sits like a stone in my stomach.

I look inside the refrigerator and find some leftover chicken salad. I wonder if it is still safe to eat and take a tentative bite.

Like everything else I try, it is tasteless, like eating wallpaper paste. I spit my mouthful out into the sink and stuff the rest of it down the garbage disposal. I make a cup of chamomile tea with honey and take it into the living room.

One wall of the living room is almost entirely glass, with a view over the neighbors' roofs to the hills beyond. Through the glass, I can see storm clouds gathering again, and this does not help my mood. There are still a few logs left in the brass bin on the granite hearth. I stack them in the fireplace grate, add some crumpled newspaper, and strike a match. I settle on the couch with my tea and the fire. Nick's pictures are still displayed on the mantel. "What should I do now?" I ask his portrait. The rain falls steadily, the fire burns itself out, and my tea grows cold as I wait for an answer that never comes.

Truth Hurts

chapter ten

The return address on the thick, white envelope says "Contra Costa Sheriff's Department, Office of the Coroner." My heart leaps. My first thought is that they must be writing to tell me that Nick is alive and they want me to come down and pick him up. I want so much for this all to be a mistake. The absurdity of this train of thought hits me one second later. In a blink of an eye, I climbed the mountain of hope and then dropped to the depths of despair. I am embarrassed by my willingness to still hope that this is all just a bad dream.

I sit and stare at the official blue printing, at my name type-written in black in the center, for almost half an hour before working up the nerve to open the envelope. Inside are five sheets, neatly stapled together. It is the autopsy report.

The first page is a typed form with basic information: "De-cedent Name," "Date of Death," "Date of Report," "Next of Kin."

"Place of Death" is listed as the hospital, although I know he was already dead when he got there. The four spaces for "Witnesses to the Death" are all blank. The police told me that this is the primary reason the autopsy was required. In legal terms, Nick died "unattended." That means that he died alone.

The next page provides a summary of findings. "Cause of Death: Sudden cardiac death associated with exercise. Due to: Atherosclerotic Coronary Artery Disease." This is followed by four single-spaced pages, astonishing in their level of detail. "The scalp hair is black with graying at the temples, wavy, and averages approximately 3 cm in length. . . . The fingernails are uninjured and clipped short. . . . On the bridge of the nose is an ovoid 1.5 cm abrasion. On the point of the chin is a 1 cm abrasion. . . ." They are just as thorough on the inside: "The right lung weighs 790 grams. . . . The liver weights 2050 grams and is covered by a smooth, intact capsular surface with sharp anterior margins."

I skip to the part about his heart, listed under the heading "Cardiovascular System." It begins: "The heart weighs 400 grams and is of the usual configuration covered by a smooth glistening epicardium with no epicardial petechiae." I read the rest of the paragraph very slowly, trying to extract some meaning from indecipherable strings of words. "All coronary arteries exhibit severe calcific atherosclerosis with segmental pinpoint luminal narrowing of the distal LAD and LCS by plaque." I can tell that this is not good. But it's only one sentence in an otherwise good report. The report continues with: "The heart valves are normally formed, pliable and intact. . . . No grossly identifiable acute infarct. . . . No recent thrombosis. . . . No aneurysm . . . . No vegetations."

I read through the report several times but still can't find a clue as to why Nick had to die.

—w—

When I was a child, we ate dinner at the same time every night, and we always sat in the exact same places at the table. Even long after we were all grown and gone, when we reassembled for holiday dinners, we naturally navigated to our old places: my father at head, my mother at foot, my older sister, Judy, and my brother, John, on one side, and my younger sister, Jane, and I on the other. Now I have family dinners with the kids most nights, but our places at the round table in the kitchen are not fixed. We sit according to shifting circumstance rather than unbending habit. I'm glad of this now because it means that no space stands waiting for Nick, or announces his absence.

"So, what did you do today?" Matthew asks me between mouthfuls.

I push the food around my plate. "I just took care of some paperwork," I say, trying to sound casual and light. "How did the day go for you guys?"

Nikolaus seems grumpy. "I walk down the hall, and everyone passing me says, 'Sorry. Sorry. Sorry.' It's like the stewardesses when you get off the plane, saying, 'Bye-bye, bye-bye, bye-bye.'"

"Everybody was saying sorry to me today, too," Matthew offered. "But I could tell that they were just glad that it didn't happen to them."

We eat in silence for a while, and then Matthew asks me, "Did you cry today?"

"No, honey, I didn't," I say truthfully. I wanted to, but I didn't.

"I'm sick of lasagna," Matthew says, poking his fork into the noodles on his plate in disgust. "Can't we have something else for a change?"

"Be thankful you've got something to eat at all," Nikolaus shoots back. He is looking at my plate, where I have carefully formed little mounds of food on each side.

I try to be conciliatory. "I guess we have had our fill of

lasagna," I say. I rise and scrape my plate off into the garbage. "Maybe tomorrow I'll make something else."

"I don't know why everyone is still bringing us food," Nikolaus says. "Are we a charity case now?"

"They are just trying to help," I say.

The phone rings.

"Maybe that's Papa," Matthew says brightly, not thinking.

"Of course it's not Papa," Nikolaus says. Matthew's face crumples quickly into a mask of sorrow and disgust. He blinks against the tears stinging his eyes.

"It's okay, honey," I say. "Sometimes I forget, too." I reach over to give him a hug, but he pulls away as if my hand were a hot poker.

"I'm done with dinner," he says and sullenly retreats to the couch and flips on the TV.

"I'll talk to him," Nikolaus says. "You get the phone."

The voice on the phone is asking for Nick Lenhart.

"Who may I say is calling?" I ask.

"Western Bank. It's regarding his credit card."

Oh, God. I think that's the one that we owe $8,000 on. Are we overdue? I try to stay calm, cool. *I can handle this. Think of what Jackie would do. Be strong.* "Mr. Lenhart is not available right now, but this is his wife. Perhaps I can help you with something?"

"Yes, Ma'am, perhaps you can. You and Mr. Lenhart currently hold our preferred Visa, and so you are entitled to several special services. If you have a few moments, I'd like to tell you about some of these now."

He is talking fast, but his words penetrate my brain slowly, like a steamship through Jell-O. It's like he's speaking a different language, and I have to take a moment to translate his message. "Are you calling about the money we owe on our card?"

"No, Ma'am!" He sounds more relieved than I feel. "I'm

calling tonight to tell you about the special services available through your current Western Bank Visa account."

For God's sake, he's not dunning me, he's trying to sell me something. "Thank you for calling," I say sincerely, and hang up.

"Who was that?" Nikolaus asks as I join the boys on the couch.

"Just a salesman," I say.

—m—

Nick was an early riser, and his first act of the day was making coffee. The aroma would permeate the house, teasing the rest of us out of our beds. I can't drink coffee now. The taste that was once so welcome now seems harsh and bitter. I hate its darkness, its pungent odor. Even the smell seems acrid, fetid.

I look over my shopping list: chamomile tea, Jell-O, milk, tissues. I'll figure out the rest when I get to the store.

The local Safeway seems different today, foreign. The lights are brighter, for one thing. The screaming packages are stacked high on endless shelves. Bands of gleaming linoleum reach out to the horizon. I'm overwhelmed—exhausted before I start.

I've shopped at this store for years, but suddenly, I can't remember where the tea aisle is or where I might find facial tissues. I am hunched over the small plastic directory on the shopping-cart seat when I feel a hand on my back. I look up. It's Claire from down the street. Claire is one of those people who are always in control, always ready to take charge. She's been president of the parents' association of our kids' elementary school several times; she is always Room Mother in her kids' classrooms and Team Mom for their sports teams. Despite her many activities, her hair is always perfectly cut, she wears just the right amount of makeup, and she favors expensive sweaters that change with the season: pumpkins in October, chicks and bunnies in April, flags in July. I admire her energy and organization, but I don't like her very much. I don't want her to see me aimlessly wandering the aisles, but it's too late to avoid her.

"Didn't Nikolaus tell you that I would go to the store for you?" she demands.

I honestly can't remember. We've had so many calls. All I can think to say is, "Gee, we've had so many calls."

"Well, I'm sure you have more important things to do than shopping," she says indignantly. Actually, since I can't seem to concentrate and my clients won't return my calls, I really don't have that much to do. But I don't contradict her. Women like Claire make me feel inadequate even on my best day, and this is far from my best day. She has a silver pin on her collar from which dangle three little hearts that no doubt represent her children. I look down and notice that the sweatshirt I'm wearing has a stain on it. She continues, "From now on, when you need something, you call me."

"Thanks," I say feebly. She nods curtly, satisfied that she's done all she can do with me for right now. I want to crawl back home and die, but I can't leave the store without at least a few basic items. "Do you happen to know where the Kleenex aisle is?" I ask.

A few minutes later I'm in line and the checkout person makes no comment as she slides ten boxes of Kleenex and a single carton of milk through the checkout. I decide to pick up fast food for dinner.

—◊—

I've just gotten back from McDonald's when the phone rings. I rush to pick it up, hoping it's Melanie returning my call with a project to offer me, along with a paycheck. But it's Ruth Miner's voice that comes through the phone. She gets right to the point: "We need to talk about Nikolaus."

"What about Nikolaus?"

"I'm going to look for an apartment near his school. That way, he can live with me until he graduates."

I think that I must have misheard her. "An apartment? Why can't he just continue to live here?"

"Well, it's just that I'm not sure what your plans are now. And I think that it is extremely important for Nikolaus to stay in the same school and graduate with his class."

"I agree. That's very important. That's why he should continue to live here."

"I know that you are probably planning to move back east and be closer to *your* family."

"I don't have any plans to move," I say through clenched teeth. "In fact, I don't have any plans at all. I just buried my husband last week. I haven't really had time to make any plans."

Ruth's tone turns saccharine. "I'm just trying to help. I thought that it might be best for you to be near your family at a time like this. And there is nothing holding you here now."

"I have my family here. Nikolaus, Matthew, and Elisabeth are my family."

"Your life may go in a different direction now. I just want to make sure that Nikolaus is taken care of."

"Nikolaus is my son. We are a family. Any plans we make will take into account what is best for him."

There is a frosty silence, and then Ruth says, "With all you have on your mind, you may not be thinking clearly about Nikolaus. He is my grandson. I just want you to know that I'm willing to do whatever is necessary for him."

"I'll certainly keep that in mind. Thanks for the call."

Honoring
Memories

chapter eleven

E ven when Nick and I were first dating, I wasn't so naive as to think that Rachael's family would welcome me with open arms. Of course, I hoped that in time, they would come to accept me. I never thought that they would still view me as an outsider ten years later.

Since her teenage years, Rachael was a "brittle" diabetic, which means that she was prone to wild swings in blood sugar that could be suddenly serious or even fatal. A critically ill child has a profound effect on a family. The child's needs naturally trump all other considerations. Every birthday, every holiday might be her last. Nick and Rachael spent every holiday with Rachael's family, never with Nick's. The Miners joined them on every vacation, just in case Rachael had an incident. Robyn and her husband, Jeff, always came along, as well. By the time Rachael died, the pattern had been long established. When Nick and I got together, however, all that was inevitably going to change.

Ruth and Robyn were suspicious of me from the beginning. The fact that Nick and I met in a somewhat unusual way didn't help matters. I was living in Atlanta, working for an ad agency. I got on a flight to San Francisco, and Nick was sitting next to me. We struck up a conversation. Rachael had died about six months before. During that flight, he talked about his work, about Nikolaus, about his relationship with the Miners, and about how grateful he was to them for all their help. Two weeks later, I was back in San Francisco for a conference, and Nick and I had dinner together. The next week, he had a business trip to Atlanta, and we had dinner again. We began having long phone conversations. We looked for reasons to find ourselves in the same city.

We'd known each other about six months when I flew out to California to meet Nikolaus and the Miners. Nikolaus and I hit it off right away. He was a sweet, loving child, and it was obvious that he desperately wanted a mom. The Miners were cordial but cold. Over the next few months, I made the decision to move out to California permanently. A little over a year after our first meeting, Nick and I were married.

To Robyn, who had married her high school sweetheart and never ventured farther than a fifty-mile radius of her Oakland home, my story was fraught with unfathomable choices, awash in incomprehensible outcomes. She didn't think much of me, and she never let an opportunity pass to let me know it.

When I moved into Nick's house, I naturally made some changes.

"I want you to feel comfortable here," Nick said. "I want this to be your home—*our* home."

"Then please pack up the wedding pictures," I asked. "And let's put away Rachael's collection of figurines."

"Where are Rachael's wedding pictures?" Robyn asked the next day when she picked Nikolaus up for a play date with her son Ryan. "And what happened to her figurines?"

"We put them away," I said. "I was afraid I would break them."

After a long moment, she said, "I see."

Later, when we were preparing for our own wedding, Nick sold Rachael's wedding china. An ad in the paper brought a young woman with stringy hair flashing a mini diamond on her left hand, trailed by her mother. "We want to sell the whole set," Nick said. "You have to take everything." They did.

When Rachael was alive, Robyn and Jeff came to dinner at least once a week, and they continued this tradition even after I moved in. I was reluctant to tell Nick how uncomfortable they made me feel—and besides, Nikolaus looked forward to seeing Ryan. "Why aren't we using the good china?" Robyn asked when she and her husband came over for dinner the following week. She was glaring at me.

There was an uncomfortable silence. Then, Nick said, "I decided to sell it."

"I'll get some more gravy," I said, and I hurried into the kitchen. I have no idea what was said in my absence, nor did I especially want to find out.

"Did you sell the figurines, too?" Ruth Miner asked the next day when she dropped off Nikolaus after picking him up from school.

"No, I packed them away," Nick answered.

"Those figurines are quite valuable," Ruth said. "I have a duty to watch out for Nikolaus's interests because they belong to him now."

Ruth had been Nikolaus's surrogate mother for all the years that Rachael was too sick to care for an infant or a toddler. When Nick and I were first married, she continued to pick up Nikolaus after school, make him snacks, and help him with his homework. I understood why Ruth was not thrilled to have another woman in Nikolaus's life, especially someone who had very little experience with children. I can't say that I blame her. In her place, I might have felt exactly the same way.

Ruth objected when Nikolaus started calling me "Mom."

"She's not your mom," she said to Nikolaus. "Your mom loved you very much, and it would hurt her to hear you say that."

She made a point of telling me that she felt his calling me "Mom" was disrespectful to Rachael and that she would not tolerate that. I didn't want to press the point, and Nikolaus returned to calling me by my first name. It felt strange to have a seven-year-old calling me Gloria, but the alternatives—Mrs. Lenhart, Aunt Gloria—seemed equally odd. Nikolaus continued to use "my mom" when talking about me to anyone except the Miners.

Nick saw the way the Miners treated me and he didn't like it.

"They need to get over it," he said. "I have a right to go on with my life. And Nikolaus deserves a chance to have a living mother. They seem more concerned with honoring Rachael's memory than with what Nikolaus needs now."

Nikolaus's grandfather, LeRoy Miner, was aware of his wife's behavior and always went out of his way to be extra nice to me. Once, when Nick and I were at the Miners' to pick up Nikolaus, Ruth was in a particularly nasty mood. She berated me for not sending Nikolaus to school that morning with a sweater. It was cold in the morning, she scolded, and Nikolaus was fragile and could easily catch cold. Nick explained that he was the one who had taken Nikolaus to school that morning and insisted that it was not cold. Ruth clearly thought that Nick was lying to hide my incompetence. Nick stormed out with Nikolaus in tow. As I trailed behind them, wondering if there were some way to smooth things over, LeRoy came up behind me and tapped me on the shoulder. He held a fully bloomed gardenia cupped in his hand. "Rachael loved these flowers," he said, handing me the fragrant blossom. "I thought you'd like them, too."

Honoring Memories

While our relationship with the Miners was rocky, our relationship with Rachael's sister, Robyn, could be described as a guerrilla war, with Nikolaus held hostage.

Every time Nikolaus came back from a play date at Robyn's house, he'd seem depressed, and each visit was worse. He'd lose his appetite, become easily distracted, and have trouble following a simple bedtime story. "Aunt Robyn always wants me to draw pictures of Mommy," he'd confide in us, "but sometimes I'd rather do something else."

Nick had several discussions with Robyn. I don't know what was said. I do know that Robyn stopped coming over to our house after that, although she still saw Nikolaus when he was visiting Ruth's home.

By that time, Nick and I were busy house hunting. Nick's house was small, with only a concrete patio in the back, and the local schools did not have a good reputation. So we looked for a house with a bigger yard, safer streets, better schools. We found one in a town about twenty minutes away. We were anxious to move before Nikolaus started first grade in the fall. As far as Ruth and Robyn were concerned, you would have thought we were rushing Nikolaus out of town and taking him to Timbuktu.

"Grandma Ruth says we shouldn't be in such a rush to move," Nikolaus told us worriedly. "She says that after we move, I won't see her anymore."

"Of course you'll see her," Nick snapped, annoyed.

I tried to assure him. "We'll drive over to see her, and she can visit us."

"She thinks that we are moving away because we're mad at her," he says.

"That's not true," Nick said. "I'll have a talk with Grandma Ruth."

"And Aunt Robyn says we should go to the cemetery to see Mommy," Nikolaus continued. "She says that me and Papa should go to the cemetery even if Gloria doesn't want to go." Actually, I had no problem taking Nikolaus to the cemetery, but Nick didn't allow it. He didn't like cemeteries, and he didn't want Nikolaus to remember his mother that way.

"I'll have a talk with Aunt Robyn, too," Nick said.

It was after those talks that Robyn stopped speaking to us entirely and Ruth became even more difficult.

Taking Charge

chapter twelve

Nick has been gone for two weeks now, but it feels like two years. With the kids back in school, I decide to stop moping and to start dealing with the new realities of my life. I need to be rational, organized. A to-do list won't work—I'm not really sure *what* to do—so I decide to make a list of issues instead. I'll figure out my first steps later. I take a blank sheet of paper, and at the top I write "Issues."

First, I write down "Nikolaus." Ruth Miner is out looking for an apartment, and Rob Miner may already be Nikolaus's legal guardian. I can't bring myself to forge Nick's signature on his will, much less ask someone to falsely witness it. That brings me to the issue of the will, and I write that down, too. "Will." Clearly I need some legal advice on the will. But that will cost money, and I already have a stack of bills I haven't been able to bring myself to look at. I write down "Money." I briefly consider adding

"Taxes" to the list, but then I decide that taxes are really a subset of "Money." Plus, I have until April to figure out our tax return, and it's only February. Plenty of time for that issue later.

I review my list: Nikolaus. Will. Money.

Only three things. I'm feeling more optimistic already. I think for a moment and then add one more item: I scribble "Health Insurance." I'm afraid we might not have any. We got our insurance through Nick's employer, and I have no idea how long his health coverage will continue.

The day before the funeral, I had gone to Mervyn's, the discount chain Nick worked for, to buy Matthew a pair of dress shoes. At the checkout, I automatically handed the cashier our employee discount card. He scanned it and then looked at the register readout with concern. "I'm sorry, Ma'am, but it says that this employee has been terminated."

Seeing my look of surprise, he reached over and laid his hand on my shoulder. "Didn't they tell you?" he asked. "How cold."

If they cancelled our employee discount before Nick was even buried, I was not at all confident about our health insurance.

When you are self-employed like I am, you have to take care of things like health insurance yourself. This is a lot easier when you have a husband with a steady income and a benefits package. Two weeks ago, I had that. Now, I'm truly on my own.

Nick's secretary, Janet, had pulled me aside at the funeral. "If there's anything I can do . . ." Janet would at least be able to tell me where we stood with health coverage.

"I was going to call you this morning," Janet says when I get her on the phone. "There are some things that I need from you. But first tell me what you are calling about."

"Health insurance," I say. "I want to know if we are still covered."

"If you or the kids need a doctor, I'm sure you're still covered, at least right now," Janet says. "But you need to talk to Darla in the Compensation and Benefits department as soon as you can. I just got a notice today asking me to confirm date of termin– . . . I mean, the, uh, effective date . . ."

"Don't worry, Janet, I know what you're trying to say," I tell her. "Maybe you could just connect me with Darla."

"I've been meaning to call you," Darla says when I tell her my name. I seem to be on everyone's call list today. "I'm sorry about your loss." She pauses for a moment, and then she says, "I wanted to set up a time with you to go over your full benefit package. When can you come in?"

Full benefit package. This sounds good. I want to ask her if a life insurance payment is included in this full benefit package, but I can't think of a way to ask that doesn't sound crass and greedy and like I'm willing to trade my husband for money.

"I'm most concerned about health insurance," I say. "Can you tell me if we are still covered?"

"Health benefits continue uninterrupted until the end of the month of termination," she says. She doesn't stumble over "termination" at all. I guess that in Comp and Benefits, termination is an everyday occurrence. "In other words, you're covered in full until the end of this month."

"That's only about two weeks," I say. "What about after that?"

"You have the option of continuing under COBRA. Are you familiar with COBRA?"

I'm not.

"COBRA is a federally mandated program that allows dependents to continue health coverage at their own expense for a specified length of time," Darla says, now on autopilot. "In a case of employee death, that length of time is three years. Your cost will be based on the premium required to maintain the same level of coverage you had during the term of employment."

Out of that whole stream, I heard only "three years" and "cost." When she pauses to take a breath, I ask, "What will it cost?"

"I can have the exact figure for you when we meet. But you can plan on about four hundred dollars."

I breathe a sigh of relief. "Only four hundred dollars a year?"

There is a moment of silence before Darla says, "The four hundred dollars is a monthly fee. Your husband had the executive-level plan that includes dental and vision care, and both of your children are covered."

This is bad news. Plus, the phrase "both of your children" ties a knot in my stomach since Nikolaus is not technically my child. Yet another reason that I have to address the Nikolaus issue as soon as possible. I make an appointment to meet with Darla and get off the phone. I have to talk to a lawyer and soon. How much will *that* cost? As usual, everything eventually comes back to the Money issue. I'll definitely have to get to work on the Money issue.

My client Melanie calls that afternoon. "How are you doing?" she asks.

"I'm ready to get back to work," I say.

"I had to call in another consultant to take on the spring campaign," she says regretfully. "There were deadlines coming up, and I wasn't sure when you'd be back. I hope you understand."

I understand completely. Melanie's projects are always fast paced and often high profile. Two weeks is an eternity in her world, and I don't blame her a bit for moving on without me. "No problem," I say. "I fully expected that you would carry on. I just wanted to call and let you know I am available if anything else comes up."

"I'll be out of town next week," she says, "but we should get together when I get back. I've got a bunch of projects on my plate, and I could use your help."

"Thanks," I say, and I mean it.

—⟋∿⟍—

During the night, when I am lying in bed, staring at the ceiling, and waiting for Nick, I have plenty of time to think. I've been trying to think of anyone I know who could recommend a good adoption lawyer. I know a few families who have adopted children, but they've adopted infants, and most of them came from overseas. They'd be great people to ask about finding an adoption agency, but their experience doesn't really apply to my situation. I know families who have gone through divorce, but none that I know well enough to share my concerns about custody of Nikolaus. Until I can get my legal standing straightened out, I don't want anyone questioning my authority to continue to sign permission slips, review school records, or, God forbid, authorize medical treatment.

One morning, after the kids are in school, I go over to Annemarie's to find out how she's doing with her divorce. I also have an ulterior motive.

"How did you find your lawyer?" I ask when we have settled in, she with a cup of coffee and I with the chamomile tea I brought from home.

"I asked everyone I knew who had gone through a divorce," she answers. "A few people said good things about Jerry, so I called him."

"Do you think he'd do an adoption?" I ask.

"I think he mostly handles divorces," she says, "but his business card says 'Family Law,' so he may do adoptions, too. Why?"

I decide to level with her. "I need some legal advice about adopting Nikolaus."

"You never adopted him? I'm surprised. I just assumed you had."

"It's really important that everyone continues to assume that. Please promise me that you won't tell anyone."

Annemarie is thoughtful. "If you haven't adopted him yet, why do it now? After all, he's nearly an adult, and you're his legal guardian."

"He's got two years before he turns eighteen. And I'm not

sure that I *am* his legal guardian. I'm not even sure that I can legally sign a field trip permission slip for him."

"But no one would question that. Everyone knows that you're his mom."

"But don't you see? I'm *not* his mom, not in the legal sense. I don't think I'm *anything* legally. And now I think his grand-mother, Ruth Miner, may try to take him away." Saying it out loud causes a lump to rise in my throat. I choke on the words.

"That's crazy. Why would she do that?"

"Because she feels that Nikolaus should be raised by fam-ily, and she doesn't see me as Nikolaus's family." I mop the tears streaming down my face with the napkin I had been twisting in my hands.

"But you *are* Nikolaus's family. You're his mom." Annemarie passes me a fresh napkin.

"Trust me. She doesn't see it that way."

Annemarie shakes her head in disgust. "And I thought my situation was bad. My major concern about divorcing Kurt is the house. It will be tough on the kids if I don't get to keep the house."

"I'm not sure I can keep my house, either."

Annemarie's eyes widen in sudden comprehension. "Oh my God. If Ruth Miner gets custody of Nikolaus, she could petition for his share of Nick's estate. That would include part of the house."

This never occurred to me. I feel the color draining from my face. "That can't be true. They wouldn't do that. They couldn't do that. Could they?" I try to take a sip of my tea, but I can't control my shaking hands.

"You need a lawyer—and fast." She stands up, walks over to the phone, and begins to punch buttons. "Let me see if I can get Jerry to see you today."

Legal Advice

chapter thirteen

The law offices are located in a cluster of one-story office buildings whose design might have been lifted from a high-end condo complex or a retirement resort. I have forgotten to ask Annemarie about Jerry's fees, but in the long run, it doesn't matter how much it costs to adopt Nikolaus. The money is beside the point—somehow, I'll manage to find the money, however much it takes. All I want to do in this meeting is find out if Jerry can handle my case. Glancing at my watch, I promise myself that no matter what, I will be walking out of there within an hour. The bill can't be more than a couple of hundred dollars for a single hour.

I give my name to the receptionist, who sits to one side of a bank of three doors. Each door has four or five names on it, and each name carries a string of initials and a brief explanation: "Financial Advisor." "Family Therapy." "Family Law Practice."

"Estate Law and Planning." If I had the money, these doors might hold the answers to a lot of my problems.

Despite working for a dozen people, the receptionist seems to have a lot of time on her hands. She is keeping busy now by getting estimates on vinyl-clad replacement windows, which, from the spanking-new look of this place, cannot be a work-related task. I am the only other person in the lobby, and she doesn't seem concerned about me. Ten minutes pass. A coffee table holds an arrangement of the most boring magazines I have ever seen: *Law Practice Today, Golf Digest, California Law Business Magazine.* Ten more minutes pass. I look through the meager selection of books that sit in a wicker basket next to a child-size table and chair. Just as I'm starting to flip through the opening pages of *It's Not Your Fault, Koko Bear,* the receptionist announces, "Mr. Carroll will see you now."

Jerry Carroll is a small man with a receding hairline, a rumpled shirt, and a nondescript tie. His office is small and utilitarian—desk, laptop computer, framed diplomas, a few well-thumbed books. He calls me Mrs. Lenhart. I call him Mr. Carroll. He gets right down to business. "I understand that you have an adoption matter to discuss."

"It's about my son. My husband died, and I'm concerned about my legal relationship with my son. You see, he's my husband's son—my stepson. I have a son, as well—that is, my husband and I do together." I've rehearsed this speech, but I'm so nervous now that I feel like I'm babbling, not making sense, not getting the story out quick enough.

He asks, "Are you looking to share custody of the child with the boy's mother?"

"His mother is dead."

"So the boy's mother is dead, and his father is now dead." He begins taking notes on a yellow pad. "How long were you and the father married?"

Legal Advice

"Ten years." He makes a note.

"When did the child's mother pass away?"

"Eleven years ago." He writes it down.

"Did the child live with you throughout your marriage?"

"Yes."

He puts his pen aside. "This is a simple case then. We can begin by filing for legal guardianship and simultaneously begin the adoption process. Assuming there are no glitches, the adoption can probably be completed for under two thousand dollars. We can begin drawing up the papers to initiate the process now if you like."

"No, wait. I'm not sure that this will be as easy as you think." I tell him about Nick's will. I tell him about Rob Miner. I tell him about Ruth Miner. He listens and then asks me to repeat each piece of information again so he can write it down.

"I'm sorry to ask you this," he says, reviewing his notes, "but it will be easier if I have all the relevant information now. Are there any possible grounds for you to be denied custody of Nikolaus? I'm thinking of things like drug or alcohol abuse, prostitution, battering, verbal abuse, felony convictions. Anything like that, either now or in the past?"

My face must have shown how repulsed I was by his list. "I'm sorry," he says, "but I have to ask," and then he waits for me to answer.

"No," I say, emphatically. "There's none of that involved."

"Is there anyone but you and the child living in your house right now? A boyfriend, a girlfriend—that sort of thing?"

"My other son, Matthew, lives with us, of course. He's six. And my mother-in-law stays for the weekend on occasion." I deliberately ignore the real question he is asking, and he doesn't pursue it.

There are more questions—where the kids go to school, what kinds of activities they are involved in, and how many times the police have been called out to our house. He asks if there are any financial reasons I might want to adopt Nikolaus—trust funds, inheritances, large sums of money that could be squandered. I wish.

"Nikolaus has a college fund, of course," I tell him. "He'll be applying to colleges next year."

"Where did the money in the college fund come from?" he asks.

"Nikolaus gets a small Social Security check because his mother died. But she didn't work very long, so it's only a few hundred dollars a month. We put that in his college fund. And there have been gifts from the family. And my husband and I added to it when we could."

"How much of the money was contributed by your son's grandparents?"

"Almost none." I thought for a moment. "Actually, not one cent of it came from his grandparents. They never gave him money. Even for his birthday or Christmas, they gave him Hot Wheels or video games, but never money."

All this talk of money suddenly reminds me of the fees I am accruing. I look at my watch. I've been in his office only forty minutes, though it seems like four hours. "So where do you think I stand?" I ask. "And where do I go from here?"

He puts his pen down and leans back in his chair. "From what you've told me, the mother's family doesn't stand a chance. The court would be very reluctant to pull a child from a good home that he is accustomed to, and where he is being raised by a stable adult in the company of a half-brother."

I suddenly realize that I had been sitting on the edge of the chair. I become aware that my hands ache from being tightly clenched. As I begin to understand that my worst fear is probably not a problem at all, I feel like a puppet whose strings have been cut. I slump back into the chair, and my body feels limp.

Legal Advice

Jerry glances down at his notes and then continues, "I also don't think you have cause to be concerned about the Miners taking financial control of your home or other assets. They could possibly ask the court to appoint them as managers of your son's college fund or any trust fund that may result from your husband's death. But if they can't prove that the college funds were accumulated from their contributions, their only recourse would be to prove mismanagement of funds. And that is difficult to do. Unless the assets in the college fund or trust were substantial, it would not be worth the legal fees to pursue it."

I am suddenly very tired. I feel like I could easily curl up in the chair and fall asleep. Instead, I stand up. "Thank you so much," I say. "I can't tell you how much better I feel."

But Jerry is not done. "From what you have told me of your situation, I believe that there is only one person who could derail your adoption of Nikolaus." He leans back in his chair and tents his fingers in a way that indicates he has a lot more to say. "As far your son is concerned, your husband's will is largely irrelevant. A will controls the disposition of property. A child is not property. A family court would view whatever is contained in the will as guidance only. And the named guardian—in this case, your son's uncle—will have to demonstrate that he could provide a better home for the child than you could. Since Rob Miner is divorced and does not have full custody of his own children, that's unlikely to happen. In fact, I doubt that he would even try. After all, not everyone wants to take on a sixteen-year-old boy." He smiles, and I have no doubt that he's thinking that he certainly wouldn't want to. His office is oddly devoid of any personal pictures. No wife, kids, dog, boat—nothing.

"What about Nikolaus's aunt, Robyn? She and her husband could provide a stable home. They have other children."

"No matter how good their home is, the court would be reluctant to take Nikolaus out of a stable home where he is being raised with his half-brother by a responsible adult. The Miners might raise objections to the adoption that could cost you time and money, but unless they can convince the court that you are an unfit mother or that your home environment is unsuitable or inappropriate for both of your sons, it is very doubtful that they will prevail."

"So who is the one person you say could derail the adoption process?"

"Nikolaus himself. Since he is over fourteen years of age, the court will ask him where *he wants* to be placed. And they will take his answer very seriously. If he wants to live with his grandparents, there will be little you can do to stop him—either legally or in fact. If I were you, my next step would be to go home and ask him what he wants to do. Then call me if you still want to pursue this matter."

—ww—

The phone is ringing as I walk in the door. It is Ruth Miner. There are a few minutes of strained chitchat before she comes to the point.

"We would like Nikolaus to come have dinner with us this weekend."

I am used to being excluded from the Miners' invitations. The unusual thing about this invitation is that she is letting me know her plans. Usually, she just talks directly to Nikolaus, and then he tells me what the arrangements are. "Sure, I guess. I don't think he has anything planned. I'll have him call you when he gets home and confirm a time."

"We want to ask him what he wants to do about his future." Her voice is friendly, but I can feel the tension underneath.

"You mean college?" I say, knowing very well that is not what she means at all.

"No, I mean the immediate future. I mean whether he would

prefer to stay with you, wherever you go, or whether he would prefer to live with us."

Immediately, I know that she must have been to see a lawyer, too. I say, "Alright, I'll have him call you."

My hands are shaking, and I want to drop the phone, but I hang on to hear her say, "We only want what is best for him. I hope you understand that." Then she hangs up.

—⚭—

When Nikolaus comes home from school, I have hot chocolate and cookies waiting. When I tell him that I need to talk to him about his grandmother, he isn't alarmed or even curious. In fact, it almost seems like he was expecting it. Still, what I tell him takes him by surprise. "Why would Grandma Ruth rent an apartment?" he asks. "Is she not getting along with Grandpa?"

"That's not it at all," I say. "She's worried about you finishing high school."

"She's thinks I won't finish high school?"

"No. She's worried that we'll move away."

"Will we have to sell this house?"

This is the big question, of course, and I'm not sure what the honest answer is. "It's too soon to know if we'll have to sell this house or not. It's been less than three weeks since . . ." I am finding it difficult to speak, but I know I need to have this conversation with Nikolaus right now. "I promise you, I will do whatever it takes to make sure that you can finish high school here, with your friends, and that you can graduate with your class. And there is money for you to go to college, so I don't want you to worry about that, either. Beyond that, you and I and Matthew together will have to decide what feels right."

"I just don't get why Grandma is renting an apartment."

I want to be frank with him, but I have to be careful what I say. Ruth is his grandmother, after all. "She wants to rent an apartment for you and her to live in. So that in case you don't want to live here anymore, you could live there with her and still go to the same school."

"But that's crazy!" Nikolaus is looking at me like I'm the one who's gone mad. "Why wouldn't I want to live here with you and Matthew? What is she thinking?"

I decide that there is no point in continuing to sugarcoat the situation. Nikolaus is old enough now that he knows what the score is. And if the Miners want to fight, it's going to be unpleasant for everyone. "You know how your grandmother and aunt feel about me. They don't like me being your mom. With Papa gone, they think it would be better if you came to live with them."

"Do you want me to go live with them?"

"Absolutely not! I don't know what Matthew and I would do without you." The minute I say this, I realize how needy I sound. My intent was to make Nikolaus feel wanted, not responsible, but it came out all wrong.

Nikolaus, however, seems relieved. "I'll talk to Grandma Ruth," he says. "Don't worry. I'll find out what's going on."

Learning
to Cope

chapter fourteen

I feel constantly surrounded by tears. Friends who call or come to visit often break down. Casual acquaintances greet us with shining eyes. People we hardly know meet us on the street and begin sobbing.

I can't face another lasagna or more fast food, so I'm back in the supermarket, determined not to leave without at least a frozen dinner. I'm heading for the freezer section when a woman I don't know accosts me.

"I heard about your husband," she says. She has tears in her eyes. "You poor thing." She throws her arms around my neck and buries her face in my shoulder. Her perfume smells familiar. I think it's a scent I wore at one time, but I've forgotten the name. I can't ask her now. She is sobbing. I have no idea who she is.

"It's okay, it's okay," I say, patting her on her back. What would Jackie do? I don't see how it can backfire on me in this case, so I say, "Thank you so much for your concern. It's nice to know that people care."

After that, I start driving to the supermarket two towns over, ten miles away, where I am anonymous.

—⁂—

I seem to cry at everything and at nothing. I cry when the mail brings more bills, when I overcook the chicken, when I find that we are out of dishwashing liquid. But my tears upset the boys, so I try to keep under control as much as I can.

Nikolaus and Matthew don't cry much, if at all. I worry about them. "I just don't feel like crying," Nikolaus says when I try to talk to him about it. "What's the point?" Matthew fights his tears back with all the strength he has. I think crying scares him. I think he is afraid to lose control. They both find other ways of coping.

Nikolaus has turned into the perfect child. He no longer has to be reminded to take out the garbage or to wipe the table after he clears it. He makes his bed, hangs up the towels in the bathroom, helps with dinner. He is also taking on "man of the house" jobs. He blows the leaves off the driveway, keeps the outside drains clear, and trims the hedges. Without my asking, he's taken on all the chores he's seen his father do. I worry about him. I wonder how long he can keep it up. Then I think that if he did go live with his grandmother, maybe he wouldn't have all this responsibility. He could be a kid again. This also makes me cry.

Matthew, on the other hand, spends all of his time playing video games. He plays one particular game constantly. It's a James Bond game, the one in which you are James Bond tracking a gang of villains through a crudely drawn warehouse. Matthew follows the barrel of his gun through a maze of hallways, picking off snipers and wiping out nests of thugs. He is becoming a very good shot, an expert. He can almost always take out the entire gang of villains without exhausting the three lives he starts the game with.

One day, we are in Target. I leave Matthew and Nikolaus in the electronics section in front of a video game set up with the James Bond game while I run through the store. When I return, Matthew is in control of the game, and three teenagers, along with Nikolaus, are watching him in awe. "Your brother is awesome on that game," I hear one of the teens say to Nikolaus.

Despite his skill in the game, I notice that Matthew seems to shoot more than is strictly necessary. As he slinks through his virtual world, his shots pockmark the walls, ricochet off the floor, and dent the metal containers that are supposed to act as shields. I've seen him simply keep shooting a wall at point-blank range until it crumbles and disintegrates. He likes to build a stockpile of ammunition and then let it all loose in a hail of gunfire that destroys everything in his path. I watch his face. He gets no satisfaction from this, no joy. He gets no relief.

Shortly before we got married, Nick put the house he lived in with Rachael up for sale. On the day of the first open house, a young Asian couple put in a full-price offer. They seemed like strong prospects, arriving at the door with a two-year-old boy in tow, the wife's belly swollen with their second child. They had a substantial down payment and had prequalified for the mortgage. They walked around the house, admiring the kitchen tile, the remodeled bathrooms, the ample closets, the tidy backyard.

As we began to finalize the sale, however, we noticed a distinct change in the couple. Suddenly they asked for more time, more inspections. They were unsure about the financing. They were worried about the neighborhood. Finally, they withdrew their offer entirely.

Nick and I were baffled by their sudden change of heart. There was nothing in the inspection reports that would sour the deal—everything checked out fine. Our realtor finally told us, apologetically, that the couple was disturbed to learn that Nick's wife had died. We protested. Rachael hadn't died in the house. She died in a hospital in San Francisco, thirty miles away. And she hadn't had a violent or unexpected death. She had been sick for a long, long time. When she died, it was, in many ways, a release. Still, the realtor explained, the couple felt strongly that Rachael's spirit may still remain in the house. This was news to us. Nick and I had been living together in that house for months with nary a light flicker or chain rattle. But we had a backup buyer, so we didn't press it any further.

I think of that couple often now. I'm sure they would say that Nick's spirit is still in this house. But as I move through the house now, willing him to come, wanting so much to see a sign of his presence, I feel nothing. I lie in our bed at night, sleepless, waiting, watching the darkness until a few hours are stolen by a dreamless sleep. By morning, only exhaustion and failure remain.

Nick was not a night person. He loved the morning. Why, then, do I expect to find him now in the darkest parts of the night? Ghosts keep their own hours. Maybe they need the alchemy of darkness to work their magic.

Matthew is restless at night, too. In the middle of the night, I'll hear his footsteps pounding down the hall, and he dives, still half asleep, into my bed. In the last hours of the night, he twists in my sheets, kicks me away. He wakes still tired and cranky. Before Nick died, this happened occasionally; now he does it almost every night.

I think a lot now of Matthew's first year. As an infant, he rarely slept through the night. Nick and I would take turns holding him, pacing the kitchen, and praying for him to calm down so we could all go back to sleep. This first year of Nick's death seems very much like the first year of Matthew's life in that I am again sleepless and exhausted. Maybe stealing sleep is a natural part of entering the world, as well as leaving it.

Looking
for Nick

chapter fifteen

Elisabeth Kübler-Ross, a physician who had done landmark research in the field of death and dying, identified five stages of grief: denial, anger, bargaining, depression, and, finally, acceptance. I think she missed a big one: pretending. I visit all the stages of grief regularly, every day. But pretending is where I live. Pretending lets me miss Nick while avoiding the crushing realization that he is completely and irrevocably gone. He's just not here right now, I pretend.

It is a sunny day, the first we've had in a long time, and I am taking the kids to the reservoir. I've packed a lunch; they have their fishing gear. As we drive through downtown, the streets look like they've been washed bright and clean by the rains and are now basking in the sunshine.

We stop at a red light. Two bikers, a man and a woman, lounge against a tree in a small, grassy square. They are dressed in black spandex shorts and bright nylon shirts. They squirt streams of water into their mouths from clear plastic bottles. They turn to look behind them, calling to someone.

Another biker is riding up the sidewalk. It's Nick. His powerful legs pump the pedals; his teeth gleam in a smile under his dark mustache. Joy and relief flood through me. I almost turn to the kids to tell them, to shout to them triumphantly, "There's Papa!" as if he's just been lost all this time. But before I can speak, the biker jumps down and slides off his helmet. The sunlight gleams on his shaved head, and I suddenly see that he is too thin, too wiry. He is not Nick.

"Go on," Nikolaus says impatiently. "The light's green."

On another day, I'm in downtown San Francisco, walking down Market Street in the noontime crowd. Up ahead bobs a head of black hair, slightly curly—just like Nick's. I know better than to follow it. I know it is not Nick. But just in case, I keep my eye on the black hair until it turns the corner and I see the proof that it is not Nick—the too-thick lips, or the swarthy skin. Look there now, across the street, a bushy mustache eats a sandwich. It's not Nick. Everywhere I see impressions of Nick—his broad shoulders, his square neck, his strong hands. But they are not Nick's. They are just physical reminders that come at me from everywhere, hit at me like a thousand fists. They are not Nick. Bits and pieces only, nothing that adds up to the whole. Not Nick. Never Nick.

I'm on the freeway, riding the middle lane, going the speed limit. I don't drive fast anymore, don't do anything fast anymore, but still, I'm inching up on the car in front of me. Looking to change lanes, I glance in the side mirror. A gray Honda is approaching in the fast lane. It's Nick's car. Nick is behind the wheel, I'm sure of it. Full head of dark hair, neatly trimmed mustache. I see him only for a second. When I look again, the car is in my blind spot. It moves alongside me, as if in slow motion, but the driver is looking away, and I can't see his face. I let him pass me and then accelerate and move behind him. I can see the outline of Nick's square headset solidly on his broad shoulders.

Nick is driving fast, as he usually does, but I'm determined to keep up. My speedometer passes seventy, then creeps past eighty. I can't afford to lose him, but I also can't risk my life this way. I am not capable of driving this fast, and Nick knows that. I ease my foot from the accelerator and let the car glide back down within the speed limit.

I'm resigned to having lost his car when suddenly I spy it a short distance ahead. He has slowed considerably and moved to the right lane. He's letting me catch up! But then, abruptly, he steers off onto an exit ramp. I must not lose him. I move into the right lane and follow him down the exit's off-ramp.

Nick's car is in the middle lane at the stop sign, his left turn signal flashing. I cut in front of another car and pull my car to a stop next to his.

The driver sits calmly behind the wheel, waiting for an opportunity to cross the two lanes of traffic in front of us. His window is open, and strains of lively Latin music drift over to my car. I see the Virgin Mary standing, firmly pasted, on the dashboard. The driver looks left, away from me, then right to face me. I see his dark olive skin, the deep cracks in his weather-beaten face. He is not Nick. He is definitely not Nick.

Bills to Pay

chapter sixteen

Having made some progress on the Nikolaus issue and the Health Insurance issue—at least, I have a meeting set—I decide to take another stab at the Money issue. It's been three weeks now since Nick died. I am sure that I can cover the next mortgage payment, which will be due next week. And I can make at least token payments toward the other bills. Beyond that, my current financial situation is like a big black hole.

The time has come for me to figure out exactly where I stand. And where I'm standing right now is in front of an enormous, disorganized heap of paperwork stacked in the corner of the upstairs office. During the awful days when I was planning the funeral, I ransacked the papers we kept in the small safe in the back of our closet to find the paperwork for cemetery plots. We used the safe to store lots of important papers: birth certificates, pink slips for the cars, insurance policies. These were all now in the pile before me. In the days before Nick died, he was preparing to do our tax return. In cleaning up before the funeral, I swept the piles of bank statements and receipts he had laid out on the dining room table and added them to this pile. All the statements and bills I've received in the past few weeks have been added, unopened, to the stack.

What would Jackie do? I wonder. Jackie had financial advisors to take care of all this stuff. Jackie never worried about paying the mortgage or the electric bill. Jackie was free to mourn her husband without being interrupted by mundane financial matters. Jackie can't help me on this one. I'm on my own.

I move my heap of papers to the center of the room and sit down on the floor beside it. My plan is to sort the paper into two piles: 1. everything I own, and 2. everything I owe. Assets and liabilities. Debit and credit. I'll start on the positive side and figure out how much money I have to work with. Then, I'll figure out the best way to spread it around to cover what I owe. At least, that's my plan.

I pick up the first paper and look at it briefly. It's a bank statement. I put it in what will become the asset pile. The next envelope contains a credit card bill. I put it in the bills pile. I notice that my hands are shaking, and I make a conscientious effort not to look at the numbers on the papers. I simply look at the letterhead and decide which pile it belongs in. Three hours later, I have created three stacks: assets, bills, and miscellaneous stuff I'm not sure what to do with. My back aches and I feel sweaty, but if I don't continue with this now, I may not have the courage to face it again later.

The asset pile is the smallest. I clear space for it on the desk and turn on the computer, then open a new spreadsheet and make careful entries for each piece of paper. There is an investment account, Nick's checking account, my checking account, and the kids' college accounts. When I've entered everything into the spreadsheet, I add all the entries and highlight the total. It's not a lot of money, but it's a better number than I thought it would be.

Then, I decide to separate the accounts I've just listed into two columns: 1. money I can get my hands on immediately, and 2. money that will be harder to access. The only account that is in the first column is the paltry sum in my checking account. This is a problem. I shuffle through the bills pile and extract three credit card bills. I take the amount shown on the "Available Credit" line of each bill and add it to my total of immediately available cash. This number looks better but would still only cover next month's mortgage payment and a few other bills.

I add up the money that will be more problematic to access: my IRA account, Nick's retirement account, the money we've been saving for Nikolaus for college, which is pretty substantial since he's only two years away, and the smaller amount we've saved for Matthew. These numbers are much more comforting, but these are emergency funds to be used only if I have no other choice.

Just to see what happens, in the immediately available funds column, I enter an amount equal to one year of Nick's salary, which is what I think Nick's life insurance policy may be worth. With this addition, my bottom line looks much healthier, and I feel much better. I decide to ignore the fact that I'm not actually sure if this money is coming through. I know Mervyn's provides life insurance for employees, but until I meet with Darla, I can't be sure how much I can count on getting or when I'll get it.

I'm feeling pretty good about things, so I decide to save my liability pile for another day. It's better to end on a positive note, and the kids will be home from school shortly. While I'm on the upbeat, I call Doug and manage to convince him to set up a meeting for later in the week.

All Business

chapter seventeen

On the forty-minute drive to Doug's office, I listen to news radio, not willing to risk a music station. Every song I hear carries a memory or an emotion, and I don't want to appear at Doug's office with a tear-stained face. Today, I'm all business. This part of my life had nothing to do with Nick. He never even met the people I work with on projects or most of my clients, so there is nothing missing here today. I am a separate entity. *I am my own person.*

Doug works for a company that provides transportation services for large construction projects around the world. If you need five bulldozers in Kuala Lumpur in order to build a power plant, they can get them there. If you need twenty-five temporary housing units placed next to a construction site to house the workers, they can do that too. They have a division that recruits skilled labor worldwide, and another division helps top executives and their families locate housing and get settled in places like Hong Kong or Budapest. They contracted with an artist friend of mine, Stephen, to design a website that would highlight their various businesses and attract more clients worldwide. Stephen brought me in to develop the content outline for the website and write the text for the site. Stephen is already in the lobby when I arrive. The last time I saw him was a few days before Nick died. We had lunch together and tossed around ideas for future projects. I like working with Stephen, but we have virtually no relationship outside of work. When Nick died he sent a huge, gorgeous floral arrangement to the house, but I don't think he came to the funeral. He had never met Nick.

Just after I arrive, we are ushered into a conference room. Three people join us: the president of the company, the vice president in charge of technology, and Doug, who is the director of marketing. We've had several meetings on this project, so I've met everyone before. Usually we greet each other with a simple handshake. Today, each one grasps my hand and holds it, strokes my shoulder, hugs me. They express their sympathy. The president of the company has tears in his eyes. The vice president asks about my kids—I didn't know they knew I had kids. They ask how I am doing. Their concern is genuine and, truthfully, very touching. But it throws me off balance. I was thinking I could come in, do the meeting, and leave all my personal issues behind. But I can't. Death invades the deepest corners of life because it touches everyone in some way.

Last night, I reviewed what I am going to present today. It's the presentation I was working on the morning that Nick died. It describes the content outline of the website. It's fairly straightforward material and I'm not expecting any controversy or major questions. I feel prepared and ready to go. I plug in my laptop and bring up the first slide. I start to explain it—a simple introduction, really—but my voice falters and cracks. On the second slide, an explanation of where we are in the project, my mind goes blank. No one but me seems disturbed by this. In fact, everyone is looking at me with sympathy.

Suddenly, I hear Doug's voice, explaining the second slide. When he finishes, I push the button, and he goes on to explain the third one, too. I struggle for something to add, but my head feels like it is full of wool. It's almost an out-of-body experience, like I'm not even in the room but floating above it, watching. I try to speak and am surprised and embarrassed when my voice squeaks out.

What's happening to me? I know what I need to say. I'm a good presenter. I can think on my feet. Now, suddenly, I can't do any of it.

The meeting starts to pick up pace. Several people are talking, adding ideas, asking questions. I can't follow what they are saying; they are going too fast. I start to panic. *Am I losing my mind?* I take a sip of the coffee that Doug has put in front of me. It tastes sour and bitter, like bile. It sloshes on the table as I put the cup down more forcefully than I intended. Stephen, sitting next to me, moves in quickly to mop up the mess. I sit there and watch him, afraid to move.

There are a few more slides, a few more questions, and then an exchange of farewell pleasantries and some hearty handshakes. Each of the others murmurs sympathies to me on the way out, and the meeting is over. Doug and Stephen stay behind to help me pack up my laptop.

"I'm sorry," I whisper, my voice still shaky. "I don't know what happened. Thanks for saving me." Stephen looks as concerned as I feel. I know he's worried that I won't be able to complete the project. I'm worried that I won't be able to complete any project ever again. I'm scared that I've lost the ability to think, to function. In fact, I'm not just scared, I'm terrified.

"It was fine," Doug says firmly. "It was a good presentation. You are not yourself yet, that's all. Give it time."

Separation
Anxiety

chapter eighteen

M y friend Barb calls to ask if Matthew can take a drive with
her family up to Tahoe for the day. Her son Kevin and Matthew are best friends. "The kids will have fun playing in the
snow," she says. I think that getting away from video games for
a day will be good for Matthew. He is not enthusiastic about the
trip, but he agrees to go.

Nikolaus is also up in the mountains this weekend. He's
with his Scouts troop on their annual snow-camping outing,
which sounds like torture to me, but Nikolaus looks forward to
it. I don't know if Nikolaus had a chance to talk to his grandmother before he left, but at least while he's up in the snow, he'll
have a respite.

"It will be good for you to have some time to yourself," Barb
says when she comes to pick up Matthew. "Read a book, go to a
movie, go shopping."

After they leave, I try to read a book, but I find myself read-ing the same sentences over and over. I get to the bottom of the page without a clue of what I've just read. I usually love to read mysteries. I like them because no matter how messy the situation is, it all gets neatly wrapped up in the end. Now when I try to read a mystery, I find that the murders really upset me. I resent the fact that everyone is so focused on finding out who did it. I want to know how the family is doing, how they are coping. Mystery stories never tell you that.

I try to watch television, but I can't seem to follow even the simplest sitcom. I forget the set-ups, and I don't get the jokes. I leave the TV on and pretend to watch it because it makes me feel more normal. It's a cover for what I'm actually doing, which is just sitting on the couch for hours, lost in my own thoughts.

Today, without Nikolaus and Matthew, freedom proves less enticing than it sounded. I drive to the mall but find little that holds my interest. The displays are filled with bright spring colors I can't imagine wearing, and the mannequins all have an attitude of aggressive happiness I could never maintain. Normally on a free afternoon, I would go to a movie, maybe something roman-tic that I know Nick and the boys wouldn't want to see. There's a movie theater in the mall, and I consider checking out what's playing. But I'm afraid that if I sit in the darkness, I'll spend the two hours crying, so I head back to the car.

The sky is slate gray, heavy with the threat of rain. Fat drops spot the windshield as I pull onto the freeway. This storm will translate into snow in the mountains. I say a small prayer for Nikolaus and Matthew to be safe.

At home, I shake off my coat and make a cup of tea. It is dark outside, although it's only three in the afternoon. I wonder if the storm will force the Scouts to break camp early. I wonder if Barb and Mike have thought to bring tire chains.

At five, I turn on the outside lights. I don't expect Barb and

Mike to be back with Matthew until six or seven, but with the storm, you never know. In the halos of light in front of the garage, I watch thick streaks of rain. Does each inch of rain translate into more or less inches of snow? I think it's more. Maybe a lot more. We've probably had two inches of rain this afternoon, so would that mean six inches of snow? The Scouts could hike through six inches of snow, and even if they were stranded, they have all the right gear with them to keep warm and dry. Still, what if this storm brought over a foot of snow, or even two or three feet? Wouldn't the weight of that much snow collapse the Scouts' snow caves, suffocating everyone inside?

I pull out the Scouts' emergency phone tree and call the person at the top, the one who would call everyone if something happened, if there were some emergency. No one answers, and I am reluctant to leave a message. There were no messages on my machine when I got home from the mall, so they probably haven't been trying to reach me. Just to make sure, I call the next number down the tree.

"Haven't heard anything," the mom who answers the phone says. "But they have enough food and gear to camp for a week if they need to. I just hope the roads are clear so they can drive home tomorrow."

These are the same roads that Matthew is on now. I wonder if Barb and Mike will decide to stay rather than risk driving home in this storm. The rain has not let up since this afternoon—if anything, it's coming down harder. I stare at the phone, willing Barb or Mike to call and say they are all safe at a motel somewhere and will be back tomorrow. I try to ignore the mental image of them with the two kids stranded in a snowdrift on the side of the road—or worse, skidding across the highway in that slow motion of accidents, spinning, spinning, glass shattering, bodies slammed against each other, against the car, against the road. The emergency road crew will find Barb's and Mike's

IDs certainly, but how will they know that Matthew is not their child? How will they know to call me? How long will I wait to hear the news until they figure it all out?

I make another cup of tea, trying to stay calm. It tastes warm and slightly metallic, like blood. I am sure that something has happened, I can feel it. When I hear the phone ring, I know it can only be someone who will confirm what I already know. I try to compose myself before I answer, but my voice shakes.

"What's wrong? You sound awful." It's Karin. I wonder why they have chosen her to tell me the bad news, and then I realize that her call has nothing to do with Nikolaus or Matthew.

"I'm waiting for a call from Nikolaus or Matthew," I tell her. "I'm pretty sure something has happened to them." I tell her my concerns about the storm in the mountains. I tell her about the tea tasting like blood. Saying it out loud makes me sound a bit crazy, but then Karin is the one person I know who has near-absolute faith in signs, in intuition. I know she'll understand.

"Relax," she tells me. "You are getting all worked up over nothing."

"Don't you think I should trust my intuition?" I say. "I feel like I know in my bones that something bad has happened."

"What were you doing the morning Nick died?" she asks.

"I was working on a presentation for one of my clients."

"Did you have any idea that he had died?"

I try to remember what I was thinking, how I felt that morning, before the neighbor came to the door, before I ran out to the ambulance, before I went to the hospital. It's hard to do. The curtain of memory between the before and after is ironclad, death's harsh glare obscuring all that went before it with a deep shadow. "I didn't even think he was dead when I first saw his body," I have to admit.

"I think you can relax then. No offense, but I don't think your intuition is all that great."

A sweep of light crosses the living room—headlights of a car in the driveway. "I've got to go now," I say. "I think Matthew's home."

"The roads weren't bad at all," Mike tells me, puzzled by the prolonged hug I'm giving Matthew. "This storm is local. It's not even snowing up in the mountains."

Financial Security

chapter nineteen

I know exactly where to go to meet Darla, my contact in Mervyn's Compensation and Benefits department. Nick worked for Mervyn's for almost ten years, and her office is in the same building his had been in.

If I were going to Nick's office, though, I would use the back lobby—the one with indoor/outdoor carpeting and plastic chairs filled with people applying for entry-level jobs and salesmen lugging sample cases. But Darla told me to come to the front lobby—the one with the soft music and teak furniture. In my denim skirt and tights, I would have melted into the back-lobby crowd; in the vast, beige expanse of the front lobby, I feel like a poor relation.

The receptionist takes my name and motions me toward the long leather couch. I take off my anorak and fold it carefully on the seat next to me, hoping that the black turtleneck I'm wearing looks at least a little sophisticated. My skirt suddenly feels too short. Jackie would have been more appropriately dressed. But Jackie had someone to do her laundry, lay out her clothes, do her hair. *Damn her.* I am desperately trying to feign a confident attitude when a young woman dressed in a fitted blue suit approaches, carrying a folder. She introduces herself as Darla and extends a manicured hand.

"Actually, I think that it might be best if we meet out here," she says apologetically. "All the conference rooms are booked, and unfortunately, my office is a small, noisy cubicle. We'll have more privacy here." She leans closer and whispers, "No one ever uses this lobby." Her red lips stretch over her even, white teeth in a smile that looks genuine. I am hoping I remembered to brush my teeth this morning.

Darla sits beside me on the couch and lays the folder on the low table in front of us, a slab of pink-veined marble that reminds me of a headstone. She opens the folder and extracts a single sheet of paper.

"Let's start with the retirement accounts," she says, handing me the paper. "You are, of course, the designated beneficiary. This itemizes the value of that account as of close-of-business last Friday."

I follow her gaze to the paper with numbers that march in neat columns across the page. I'm having trouble making sense of the numbers. Darla scoots closer and points to the bottom row. "As you can see, this account is now largely invested in company stock. You might want to diversify, but, of course, that's up to you. We will send you a package of instructions detailing the procedure for changing the allocation. This is just a summary of the recent totals."

"Yes, right." I nod dumbly and hand the paper back to her. She replaces it in the folder and selects another.

"This details the health benefits available to you," she continues, pointing to the new sheet. "As we discussed on the phone, you can continue coverage for up to three years. The monthly premium is $426. If the premium is not paid by the tenth of the month, your coverage will be automatically cancelled." Again, she leans closer and lowers her voice. "You can probably shop for a better rate. But at least you'll be covered in the short-term."

She reaches over, takes my hand, and gives it a brief squeeze. It happens so fast that for a moment I'm not sure that it happened at all. I realize that she is trying to help me. I decide to trust her.

"I'm concerned about health coverage for my son Nikolaus." My voice falters. "He's not really, officially—that is, legally—my son. I'm wondering if he's still eligible."

Darla lowers her mascara-thick lashes, thinking. "Do you claim him as a dependent on your tax return?"

"Yes, of course. I—that is, we—have been. I don't know what will happen this year." I feel a small trickle of cold sweat inch down my back. The Tax Return issue. I hadn't even thought about the Tax Return issue.

Darla pulls a pad of lined yellow paper from inside the folder and makes a note. "I'm pretty sure he'll still be covered," she says, "but I'll check on it."

A speaker set in the acoustic tile ceiling above us is infusing the room with a soft instrumental version of "Send in the Clowns." The backs of my knees feel damp, and I am beginning to worry that there will be a pool of sweat on the leather couch when I get up.

Darla is studying other papers in the file. She lines three of them up across the pink marble. "Let me give you a summary of the insurance and other payments that are coming to you." She flips to a clean sheet of yellow paper, tipping the pad toward me so that I can watch her write. "First, there is the insurance. All executive-level employees are automatically covered for a minimum amount. Your husband paid the premium to increase that coverage." She writes a series of neat, round, evenly spaced numbers on the first line in black felt tip.

"Then there is deferred compensation. Unfortunately, we will now have to pay it out to you in a lump sum."

I don't ask why this is "unfortunate" but simply watch as she prints another series of no-nonsense numbers under the first. My shirt is sticking to my back. Above us, a thousand violins are now playing "Stand by Your Man."

"Your husband also had options to purchase company stock at a reduced rate. About half can be exercised now, and the rest will vest over the next three years." Again, I have only the vaguest idea what she is talking about. She adds a third series of numbers to the two already on the yellow pad. "This stock option number is only an estimate, of course. It will vary depending on the stock price at time of exercise."

"Of course," I say, putting my hands under my legs.

She draws a bold, black line under the column of numbers on the pad and then carefully adds them. She writes the sum not in the small, neat numbers she used above the line but instead makes it large and bold, numbers that disregard the lines and shout out from the paper. She admires the result. I am sitting on my hands, surreptitiously trying to assess the puddle under my knees. She lays the paper in my lap triumphantly. "This is a summary of what you have coming to you."

I stare down at the sprawling, black number, the one below the line. It's a big number, bigger than I had anticipated. "Is this money?" I ask. I blink and look at it again. "Does this number represent dollars?"

Darla smiles. "Yes, it's dollars," she says. "It's your money."

The big, black number pulsates against the yellow paper. The numbers represent money. It's enough money to pay off the credit cards. Enough money to keep the house and pay the bills for years. Enough money to pay a lawyer to help me sort out what's best for Nikolaus. The pink marble is swirling. I stand up abruptly, and the paper falls to the floor.

Darla picks up the yellow paper with the big, black numbers and puts it in the folder. Then she puts the folder firmly in my hands. My legs are shaking. "This should be all the paperwork you need. Look through it when you have a chance. Don't hesitate to call me if you have questions." She takes my arm. "You seem shaken. Are you okay to drive? You can sit here for a moment if you like."

I shake my head. "Got to go now," I mumble.

I feel her grip on my arm tighten. "I'm very sorry for your loss," she says, "I didn't know your husband. But I know that he made sure you and your children were well taken care of." She lets go of my arm and looks away for a moment. "You are lucky. He must have loved you very much."

Her face is sad. I don't think it's because she's sad for me.

"I'll check on the health insurance coverage for your son and call you," she says. We are in front of the double glass doors, and she has her hand on the bar that opens it. "This is the first time I've done the paperwork for someone who has died," she says. "I have a son. He's six, just like your younger son. I'm divorced now. I wonder what would happen to him if something happened to me." She looks out at the parking lot briefly and then back at me. "I guess I better find out."

I grasp her hand and hold it a moment. "Good luck," I say, "and thank you."

I sit in my car in the parking lot for a long time. I don't have to take the yellow paper out of the folder to see the numbers dancing in front of my eyes. Money has been a big worry. But now, magically, I have money. I realize that the new state of the Money issue can help solve the Nikolaus issue, and probably lots of other issues. I start the engine and drive slowly out of the parking lot. I'm not thinking about where I'm going; I automatically head downtown. My thoughts are racing. What should I do first with the money? Pay off the credit cards? Pay down the mortgage? No, Nick had said a million times that the mortgage is the only tax break we get. Nick would know what to do with the money. Without thinking, I pick up my cell phone and speed dial Nick's number at work. He will be so excited about the money. He'll know exactly what we should do first.

I listen to Nick's number ring through as I stop at a light on Montgomery Street. It is lunchtime in the financial district, and the intersection in front of me is teeming with people. I hear the phone click through to a recorded message. "The number you have reached is not in service at this time. . . ."

The realization of what I'm doing smacks me between the eyes like a baseball bat. I drop the phone in my lap as I blink through the windshield at the stream of humanity in front of me—black, white, Asian, blond, brunet, and redhead, in every conceivable variation. Every one of them is a unique genetic combination; none of them have the combination that adds up to Nick. From now on, no matter where I go, no matter how big a crowd of people I look in, I will never find him. He isn't at work, he isn't at home, he isn't on the planet.

I don't know how long I've been sitting there before I notice the bicyclist tapping on my window. "Are you all right?" he shouts over the blaring car horns. I nod. "You better get moving before there's a riot," he says over his shoulder as he rides off.

A Whole
Different Planet

chapter twenty

D oug calls. "Can you come to a meeting tomorrow at three
o'clock?"

I had handed in the first-draft copy for his company's website over two weeks ago and was wondering when he would get
back to me with comments and revisions.

"I need you to meet with some field guys," Doug continues.
"They are usually scattered all over the country, so it's unusual
to catch them all in the home office at once. I was hoping you
wouldn't mind the short notice."

"No problem." It isn't like I had much planned, and the billable
hours would be welcome. "What will the meeting be about?"

"We'll be talking with the top sales managers to get their
thoughts and ideas on the website. The truth is, these guys won't
have any useful feedback, but they have a lot of political clout in
the company." Doug knows me well enough to tell me the truth.

"Sounds great. I can't wait," I deadpan. With Doug, I can be sarcastic.

"As far as technology goes, these guys are dinosaurs," Doug tells me. "They have their secretaries print out paper copies of their emails and then file them. The only time they'll see the website is when we show it to them. But I need to cover my rear by showing it to them now, before it's complete. All I need you to do is look interested and jot down whatever they say."

"Look, Doug, I know I messed up the last meeting. But I'm fine now. I promise I won't let you down."

"I'm not worried about you at all." Doug says, although I'm sure he's lying. "And anyway, this meeting is a piece of cake."

The next morning, I remind Matthew that he is to go to the after-school care program, and I will pick him up from there. "I may not be there until after five," I tell him, "so if you finish your homework, you'll have some time to play." I keep my voice light and cheery, but Matthew's face remains gloomy. He used to go to the after-school program several times a week, but since Nick died, he's gotten used to me picking him up right after school. "Come as early as you can," he grumbles.

I arrive at Doug's office at 2:30, hoping to catch him before the meeting and work out a presentation strategy. At 3:30, I'm still sitting in the lobby. "Sorry," the receptionist says. "The sales meeting is running long. But they should be wrapping up soon."

It is 4:10 by the time I am ushered into the conference room. A caterer is clearing the remains of sandwich platters and soft drinks. Doug greets me apologetically. He is wearing a suit and tie. I've never seen him in a suit and tie before—he's more of the khakis-and-polo-shirt type.

Doug introduces me to three men seated around a table. Everything about them says *strictly business*, from the stripe of their ties to the courtly way they call me Ms. Lenhart. I assure them that it's fine to use my first name. I'm grateful to Doug for giving me a heads-up on dressing more formally than I normally do.

"I'd like to start by giving you a quick overview of our planned website," Doug begins. "Gloria has been consulting with us on it. I've asked her to sit in with us today so that she can hear your comments and suggestions firsthand."

I nod and smile, inwardly relaxing. All Doug wants me to do is listen and take notes. *Piece of cake.*

Doug is about fifteen minutes into the presentation when I hear a buzz in my briefcase. It's my cell phone. Only a few people have my cell number: the kids, their schools, and Matthew's after-school program. I should have turned it off before the meeting started, but I didn't dare. What if something happens and the kids need to reach me?

"Is that your cell phone ringing?" one of the men asks me.

"Yes," I admit. "I'm sorry, but I'll have to excuse myself for a moment to take this call."

I dig the phone out of my briefcase and step out into the hall. "Mrs. Lenhart?" a woman's voice said. "This Katie from the Roadrunner After School Club." My heart leaps to my throat. Matthew. "Is everything okay?" I ask, trying to keep my voice steady.

"Everything is fine," the voice says. "Matthew just wants to talk to you. Would that be okay?"

"Of course. Put him on."

"Hi, Mom." Just hearing Matthew's little, sweet voice settles my heart back down.

"Hi, sweetie. Is everything okay?"

"I think I might be sick. Can you come get me soon?" He seemed fine this morning, but kids can come down with something in minutes. Or he could just be looking for attention.

"Are you really sick? Or do you just want me to come get you?"

"I might be sick. I'm not sure."

"Well, why don't you ask the Roadrunner ladies to let you lie down, and I'll be there as soon as I can, okay?"

"Okay, Mom. I love you. I'll see you soon."

The Roadrunner lady comes back on the line. "I don't think he's really sick," she whispers, "but he seemed worried about you. He insisted on calling."

"That's okay," I say, relieved. "He can call me anytime."

I slip back into the meeting. Doug is about halfway through his presentation. Not more than ten minutes pass before my briefcase is buzzing again. "Excuse me again," I murmur as I get up to leave. "She must be in great demand," I hear one of the men say caustically as I close the door behind me.

Matthew's voice comes on directly this time. "Are you alright, Mom?" he asks.

"Of course. I'm fine. Is there something wrong?" I try not to let him hear annoyance in my voice.

"No. I just called to tell you I wasn't really sick. I just miss you. Are you sure you are alright?"

"I'm fine, honey, really. I'll call you when I'm leaving here, okay?" I think about the night I waited for him to return from the snow with Barb and Mike. Is Matthew worrying about all the bad things that can happen to me when I'm not with him? Is he picturing me lying on a freeway right now?

When I return to the room, the three men are in the midst of a discussion about a sales procedure. "Is everything alright?" Doug whispers. I nod and smile.

One of men says pointedly, "While you were out of the room, we've just been reviewing the procedure for overseas sales. It's important that you understand how it works. . . ."

My phone is buzzing again. I know that it's Matthew, but there is no way I can ignore it. "I'm so sorry," I say. "It's my son. I'm afraid he's having some separation issues. I'll just be one more minute."

"I'm so sorry, Mrs. Lenhart," the Roadrunner lady says. "Matthew just insisted on calling you again."

"Put him on," I say.

"Where are you, Mom?" Matthew asks.

"I'm in a meeting, Matthew. If you stop interrupting me, I can finish the meeting and come pick you up."

"Are you going to be driving on the freeway?"

"Yes, I will. That way I can get back to you really fast."

"You won't get in a car accident?" See? I knew what he was thinking all along. I do have intuition, after all.

"Don't worry, sweetie. I'll be safe. I'll be there soon."

"I promise not to call anymore if you promise to be careful on the freeway."

"I promise. I'll see you soon."

When I return to the meeting room, the three men look stricken, shaky. Something must have happened while I was gone, and I look to Doug for a clue.

"I've explained the situation," he says.

"Oh," I say, like I know exactly what he means, even though I don't.

"We are so sorry to hear of your loss," one of the men says, and I realize that Doug has told them about Nick. "Please accept our sincere condolences."

"And you have children," another says. "How are they getting along?"

I explain that although my youngest seems to be having separation anxiety, he's a good kid and I'm sure he'll be fine. They ask about my older son, if his grades are suffering, if his college plans are now in jeopardy. Then they ask about me, how I am coping? Did I receive an insurance payment, will I have to sell my house? They ask personal questions in such a sincere, caring way that I can't help but be touched. I also realize by their questions that they are thinking of their own wives, their own children, wondering what would happen if they were in our place.

It is clear that any discussion of business is over. I finally apologize for having to leave and bring the meeting to a close. They seem reluctant to let me go. Doug says he'll walk me to my car, and the men nod agreement. There is a moment when I think they are going to hug me, but, thank God, they don't.

"I've never seen those guys so shaken up," Doug says as he loads my laptop in the trunk of my car. "It's like they think they might be next."

"Believe me, I'm getting used to people acting strangely. It happens all the time now. It's like I'm in some kind of weird state."

"It's not just a state," Doug says. "You are on a whole different planet."

Set in Stone

chapter twenty-one

The cemetery where I buried Nick is about twenty miles away from our house. There are cemeteries that are closer, but Nick had bought three plots in this cemetery when Rachael died because it was convenient to where they lived then, and close to the Miners. Two months after Rachael died, Nick buried his father in the second plot. And now Nick is buried in the third.

Entering the large, iron gates of the cemetery, you turn your back on Kmart, McDonald's, and car dealerships that line the other side of the street and enter another world—a quiet, timeless expanse of mown grass, curving paths, and stone benches. The main mausoleum, built in the early 1900s, stands at the back of the property. It is a marvel of intricately carved limestone and granite set high on a platform of white marble steps. The twelve apostles look down on visitors who climb up to enter through the impressive wooden doors. In the 1980s, they tore out the rose garden that was originally in front of the mausoleum. At the time Rachael died, they were just beginning to sell the plots. Nick bought one for Rachael and, because he knew the section would sell out fast, he bought two additional plots behind her grave. The Miners own the two empty plots next to Rachael's grave. I've always wondered why the Miners didn't take the two plots behind Rachael's grave and let Nick have three plots in a row, but what's done is done, and asking Nick about it when he was alive would have stirred up our animosity toward the Miners.

In the days before the funeral, Nick's cousin Tom and I went to the cemetery to make the burial arrangements. I hadn't been there in years, since Nikolaus was small. Nick didn't like cemeteries and seldom brought Nikolaus to visit his mother's grave. Tom parked in front of the mausoleum and we located the plots fairly easily, just a half-dozen spaces from the road.

Nick's empty plot was located directly behind Rachael's grave and next to his father's. Tom and I had brought two dozen red silk roses to decorate their two graves, but we decided not to disturb the arrangement that topped Rachael's stone, consisting of daisies topped with a pinwheel and a pink plastic teddy bear—no doubt the work of Ruth or Robyn. Instead, we arranged the flowers in the two vases embedded at the base of Nick's father's grave, where Elisabeth would eventually lie with her husband. The black headstone reads: "Nikolaus" at the top and has room for Elisabeth's name to be added later. It felt right to me to bury Nick here, next to his father and final resting place of his mother. I would have a place where I could mourn my husband and Nick's double-vaulted plot would leave open the option, depending on where life might take me, to lie with him when my time inevitably comes.

In the cemetery office that day, a woman in a dark-blue suit flipped though a file drawer of ivory index cards. "Plot

42-A," she murmured, pulling a single card and placing it on the counter in front of us. "Owner, Nikolaus Lenhart, Jr. Person to Be Buried, Unnamed."

"I'd like Nick buried there," I said.

Tom nodded. "I think that would be fine."

I might have buried Nick in the same plot with Rachael if there were no other choice. But since we already owned another empty plot, I decided to use it. Nikolaus's parents' graves would be head to head. It was an easy solution to a difficult problem.

"Only pillow monuments are allowed in the Crucifixion section," the cemetery lady told us. These are small, rectangular slabs that sit on top of slightly larger bases. Tom and I walked through a display of them on the way back to our cars. There were open-book designs, intertwined hearts, praying hands. There was a selection of cross designs: standing crosses, leaning crosses, crosses draped with a shroud. Banners could be added that proclaim Mother, Father, Daughter, Son. There were designs with the Virgin Mary and designs with a Sacred Flaming Heart.

I didn't like any of them.

"We don't have to pick the headstone today," Tom said. "Maybe it's better if you wait a while and think about what you really want."

But now, less than three months later, every time I see Elisabeth, she asks me about the headstone. It is becoming clear that there will be no peace in this world until her son is resting comfortably under a slab of granite.

I don't want to make a quick decision. Somehow, having Nick's name carved in stone seems too final. Elisabeth sees a headstone as a tribute to Nick's life. I see it as a half-ton proof of his death.

One day, I look in the phone book under Headstones. Just above the Health Club heading, in the middle of a spread of pumped-up people with six-pack abs and perfect teeth, a single line of type reads: "Headstones, see Monuments." Monuments. That seems even more portentous. If I can't bring myself to select a simple headstone, how could I hope to build a monument?

—⚒—

On Sunday, we take Elisabeth out to dinner. Afterward, we go to the cemetery. "When are you getting Nicky's headstone?" Elisabeth asks.

"Soon," I answer.

As usual, Elisabeth is not willing to drop it. "You can buy them here at the cemetery. That's where we bought the one for my husband. They have them over by the office."

"Tom and I looked at those, but I didn't like any of them," I say. I'm trying to be patient but not doing a very good job. "We'll look at them some other day. Not today."

"I think Nicky should have a headstone," Elisabeth insists.

"He will," I say forcefully enough, I hope, to end the discussion. "But not today."

As I drive through the winding road leading to the mausoleum, I realize what lies before me. This cemetery is the biggest headstone showroom in town! I'm not limited to the paltry selection Tom and I had seen at the cemetery office. Here are several hundred examples of headstones on display, in all colors and combinations, no two exactly alike. What better way to shop for what I want?

But first I park on the road nearest to Nick's grave and unload three dozen red silk roses, enough flowers for all three graves—Nick's, his father's, and Rachael's, too, if Nikolaus decides he wants to leave them for her. Matthew refuses to leave the car. Nikolaus holds his grandmother's arm as they make their way slowly to the gravesite. Even though Nick never tended to his father's or Rachael's graves, I feel that it honors him to take over this task now that he is gone. I've brought a plastic vase that we can sink into the ground to mark Nick's grave until a headstone decision is made.

As Nikolaus and Elisabeth fuss over the graves, removing the old flowers and arranging the new ones, I let Nikolaus decide which ones he wants to put on his mother's grave. Nikolaus removes the faded daisies from his mother's grave but keeps the pinwheel, arranging some roses around it. The plastic teddy bear has disappeared. I leave them to their work and wander off through the adjacent rows to do some headstone browsing.

Most inscriptions are, frankly, uninspired: Name and date. Beloved Mother. Dear Father. Loving Husband. Rest in Peace. Quite a few look like direct copies of the cemetery's display units. Light-gray granite must be the least expensive stone; it is by far the most popular. I find myself feeling sorry for the people who lie under these mass-produced stones, not because they are dead but because so little trouble seems to have gone into remembering them.

A few rows over from Nick, a polished black stone is carved to look like a big, open book. One page of the book says, "Dominick, Beloved Husband and Devoted Father," along with two dates. The other side says, "Maria, Dear Wife and Loving Mother," with only a birth date. Dominick died two years ago at age seventy-eight. Maria is now seventy-five. The grave looks lovingly tended—the grass is clipped neatly back from the base, and an arrangement of fresh flowers overflows from an urn set into the top. This polished black stone tells the story of their lives, succinctly and indelibly. Maria and Dominick probably married young, as people of their generation were inclined to do. They have children who are now middle-aged. It was a long marriage and undoubtedly a happy one. She depended on him, and he depended on her. *She misses you, Dominick,* I think. *Even now, she still takes care of you.*

I wonder what story Nick's headstone will tell. What story do I *want* it to tell? He was loved. He was taken from us too soon. We miss him terribly. Suddenly, I am so glad that I didn't bury Nick in the same plot with Rachael. I'm glad that he has his own plot. I don't know what Nick's headstone should look like, but I can't imagine carving the story of his life into Rachael's slab of pink granite. And I want to be the one who makes the decision about whether his grave is decorated with daisies and pinwheels or red roses.

I see Nikolaus and Elisabeth heading back to the car, and I hurry to join them. Matthew has fallen asleep in the back seat.

Across the road from the cemetery exit, two monument companies stand side by side. One looks like a car dealership, with a display of stones laid out behind large plate glass windows. The other looks like a small cottage that happens to have a front yard crammed with headstones. Neither is open on Sunday.

"We should stop and look at those headstones," Elisabeth gripes, expecting me to say no because I've already told her that I don't want to look at headstones today. But I'm in shopping mode now, so I pull a U-turn and park in front of the cottage. Headstones stand in tight rows in a grassless yard behind a low fence that Nikolaus easily steps over. Matthew, now wide awake, follows, looking guiltily over his shoulder, seduced by the adventure of trespassing. I stay with Elisabeth on the sidewalk, but we can still see the whole display.

Even though there are fewer headstones here than in the cemetery, there is a much wider selection of designs. In addition to the now-familiar crosses and hearts, there are roses, redwoods and pine trees, grazing deer, proud elk, praying hands (some with rosary beads), chalices topped with communion hosts, and oak trees. "Papa liked to sail," Nikolaus suggests, pointing to a sailboat skimming across one stone.

"Who would put clapping hands on a cemetery stone?" Matthew asks, pointing to a design with two hands touched together.

"I think they are supposed to be praying hands," I tell him. He has a point, though. They do look like they're clapping.

Matthew shakes his head, indignant. "I think it's really rude to clap when someone is dead," he says.

We discuss the various options without coming to a decision. Elisabeth wants a picture of Nick on the headstone. Matthew definitely does not want clapping hands. Nikolaus says he's okay with whatever everyone else wants.

I want to continue to procrastinate, and so that's what I do.

Getting Help

chapter twenty-two

Nikolaus comes back from dinner at the Miners' looking more sad and worried than I've ever seen him. "How did it go?" I ask him. He just shrugs and walks away. I don't want to press him to talk. I don't want him to be in the middle between me and the Miners, but that's where he seems to be, and I don't know what to do about it.

I am also worried about Matthew. He's seems angry a lot of the time. Specifically, he seems angry at Nick. I notice that whenever someone begins to talk about Nick, Matthew finds an excuse to leave the room. He will avoid going into the living room, which is still filled with pictures of Nick. "We should put those pictures away now," he says one day. "Papa's gone."

I'm afraid that the few memories Matthew has of Nick will get lost and all he will be able to remember is this awful anger and hurt. I'm afraid that later, when Matthew is older, he will not be able to remember anything about his father.

Someone has given us an activity book designed to help children who have experienced the death of a parent. Matthew will have no part of it. When I offer to help write down what he remembers about his papa, he presses his lips together until they turn white. He scribbles on the pages where he is supposed to draw pictures of activities he and his father liked to do together. One day, I find the book hidden in the bottom of the kitchen garbage can.

"Leave him alone," Nikolaus advises. "He'll remember what he wants to remember." I remember Nikolaus as a small boy coming home from his Aunt Robyn's house and stuffing the pictures she made him draw of his mother far under his bed. I decide to take his advice.

The counselor from Nikolaus's school calls me. "Would you like to come in and talk to me?" she asks. "I have some resources that you may find helpful." I wonder if she thinks Nikolaus is having problems adjusting, if she knows about the adoption problems. We set a time to meet.

The counselor meets me in the school office and then leads me to a large classroom crowded with metal desks. In the corner is a small room with real walls and a door that closes.

She is a thin, red-haired woman with a kind face. "Call me Sara," she says. "I'm sorry for your loss. I was wondering if I might be of some help."

Her office is tidy but cozy, with bookcases lining two walls and a rag rug on the floor. We sit not at her desk, which is pushed to one side, but at a central table with swivel chairs upholstered in a cheerful print. On her side of the table sits a small pile of books and a thin, neat folder, which she is now consulting.

"I met with Nikolaus for the first time when he returned to school after the funeral," she continues. "Then we met again last week. He seems to be adjusting well—that is, as well as can be expected. I was wondering if you are noticing any problems at home."

"We are dealing with a lot of issues right now, as you might expect," I say. "But the kids seem to doing okay, I guess. They play a lot of video games."

"That's understandable," she says. "When the real world gets scary, it's natural to want to retreat into a fantasy world. And a fantasy world that has a controller is especially appealing."

"Maybe I should try it," I reply lightly.

Her smile is warm. "I'm not sure if you are a person who finds books helpful," she says, "but I've pulled some from our counselor's collection that you may find useful." She pushes the small stack of books toward me. The titles look interesting. *Losing Someone You Love*, *Helping Children Cope with Grief*. I thank her sincerely.

She pulls a sheet of paper out of the folder and lays it in front of me. "I've called a number of community service organizations to find out what types of grief services they offer. I made this list." She points to each name in turn and provides a brief explanation of what kind of services the organization provides, who its sponsors are, and what the costs might be. I am touched and grateful that she had done this for us.

"Nikolaus seems like a very nice kid," she says. "And in my job, unfortunately, I don't have a whole lot of time to spend with the nice kids. I really think Nikolaus will be fine, but there is one thing you should know. He is very worried about you."

"About *me*? Why, what did he say?"

"Whatever he tells me is confidential, of course. But I can tell you that the best thing you can do for him right now is to try to take care of yourself. If I can help you identify resources to do that, please don't hesitate to call me."

—m—

One of the names on the list is a family counseling service, and the first thing I do when I get home is call them. They set up an appointment and fax me some preliminary paperwork that asks for our names, ages, nature of the problem, and annual household income. Three days later, the boys and I are standing in front of a large house off a main street in Oakland. A small sign discreetly announces it as the ANN MARTIN CHILDREN'S CENTER.

Nikolaus's counselor had told me that it was a nonprofit group that specialized in helping children. When I called to make the appointment, the woman on the phone explained that they offer their counseling services on a sliding scale to children who are victims of or who have witnessed violence, children with parents in prison, or children, like mine, who are dealing with loss.

"I'm not going in," Matthew announces from the back seat. "I'll just wait here."

"Come on," Nikolaus says. "Let's just get this over with."

It is a bad start. We finally coax Matthew inside, but I have to drag him up the steps. In the waiting room, he refuses my offer to read him a book or to play with the toys scattered around the room. He sits, arms crossed, on a chair in the corner of the room farthest from where Nikolaus and I sit. "Why don't you just smack him?" Nikolaus suggests.

Our counselor is young, very pretty, and painfully sincere. Her name is Adrienne. She dresses comfortably in a slightly more polished version of the khakis and fleece vests that Nikolaus always wears, and I can tell immediately that they will develop a rapport. I don't have the same hope for Matthew; he's clearly not ready to talk to anyone yet.

We spend this first session getting out the basic facts: what happened, how we felt then, how we feel now. Nikolaus and I take turns talking, adding our perspectives and finishing each other's thoughts. Matthew refuses to talk. He turns his chair away from us and stares hard out the window. I think he wants to put his hands over his ears but doesn't dare. The hour goes by, and we make appointments for each of us to see Adrienne individually within the next few weeks.

Falling Apart

chapter twenty-three

I am beginning to question whether I can stay in our house, not only from a financial standpoint but for maintenance reasons, as well. I had always viewed my house as a safe haven, but now it's beginning to betray me.

There is an odd flapping noise coming from the heat vent in the living room. After ten years in a house, you come to know what to expect, but this was new to me. I climb into the crawl space and look at the furnace. No clue there. I wonder if I should turn the heat off. What if something is seriously wrong? What if the furnace is spewing carbon monoxide into the house? I wish I knew more about heating systems. When I go back upstairs, Nikolaus has taken the cover off the vent and is holding a shredded air filter. "Do we have any extra filters?" he asks. "This one is shot."

A strong wind blows away a section of the gutter from the top of the house. Nick would have banged the twisted piece back into shape and climbed up to reattach it. I know quite a bit about fixing things—although Nick did most of the actual work, you can't stand around holding tools for ten years and not learn something. But in this case, my confidence fails me. I can't manage to carry the long, heavy ladder it would take to reach the broken section, and even if I could get it into place, I don't feel steady enough to make the climb. I look in the phone book, trying to remember which gutter company we used before. There was one we used that did a good job and there was one Nick had warned me never to call again. If I could conjure his spirit now, that's what I'd ask—not if he missed us, not what heaven was like, but which gutter company I should call.

"I'll go up to fix the gutter," Nikolaus says determinedly, but I refuse to let him, not willing to allow him to risk the two-story climb I am afraid to make myself. I drag the fallen gutter piece from the yard and hide it in the garage. Out of sight, out of mind.

The garage is a jumble of balls, bikes, plumbing parts, electrical wire, and mysterious power tools. One Saturday morning, when Nikolaus is off with his friends and Matthew is down the street at Kevin's house, I decide to try to clean it up. I survey the piles of stuff, wondering where to start. I see something odd at the bottom of one pile, and as I bend down to get a closer look, a broom handle pokes up, straight into my left eye.

A sharp sting shoots through my brain and out the back of my head, simultaneously alerting every other nerve in my body to begin screaming in unison. Grabbing my eye, I flail wildly through the garage, scraping my shins on the bike chains, knocking over a vacuum cleaner, which falls on my foot, wading blindly through unseen detritus, and searching for the way out. I cannot open my injured eye, and I cannot stop the screaming pain. *Ice,* I think. *Must get ice.* Making my way up the front stairs, stumbling into the kitchen, fumbling with the ice tray, stopping to scream, writhing in unendurable agony. Ice wrapped in a kitchen towel, pressed to my eye, cold pain now. Am I bleeding? The towel is white, clean. No blood.

I try to open my injured eye, wondering if I can still see. The pain is so intense I can't keep it open long enough to find out. I better get to a doctor. How? Can't drive. Annemarie is gone for the weekend. Call Barb. Pray that she's home, that she and Mike haven't taken Matthew and Kevin out somewhere. Phone is busy. A sign that someone's home, at least. Pressing the towel-wrapped ice to my eye, I flee out the front door, down the driveway.

Barb and Mike live two blocks away. I'm running, moaning, towel pressed to my face, tears streaming down my face, bent on getting to Barb's house as fast as I can. I pass neighbors in the midst of their Sunday-morning routines—tossing a football, washing the car, planting bulbs. They turn to look as I run past. *Poor thing,* they must be thinking, *she's finally having a breakdown.* I don't stop to correct them.

Matthew and Kevin are playing in the front yard. "What's wrong, Mom?" Matthew asks, voice panicked.

"Get Kevin's mom!" I yell, though I had wanted to seem calm.

Mike stays with the kids while Barb drives me to the optometrist, who extracts my contact lens, still intact, and determines that there is no serious damage. I get a prescription for the pain, and Barb drives me back home. Nikolaus is home by then, and Mike brings Matthew home, along with a container of soup. The boys heat the soup, replenish my ice pack, and forego their favorite TV shows to put on channels they think I'll like.

It is almost a week before I can see well enough to trust myself to drive. Nikolaus can walk to school, but I have to ask Barb to take Matthew. Annemarie gives me a ride to Safeway when we run out of milk. "I should take my driver's test," Nikolaus says. "Then I could help you." I've forgotten all about his driving test. I haven't taken him out to practice driving in weeks. Other kids are anxious to drive so that they can drive to the mall or to the movies. Nikolaus is only thinking about taking me to the super-market and Matthew to school. Again, for a terrible moment, I wonder if Ruth Miner is right. Maybe Nikolaus would be better off with her, where he wouldn't feel the weight of these responsi-bilities. Where he would be free to be a kid again.

—⁓—

As the weeks wear on, Matthew becomes increasingly sullen and withdrawn. He's had a few meetings with Adrienne, but he re-fuses to talk to her. "He'll come around," Adrienne assures me. "Just give him time."

He seems tired all the time, though he gets plenty of sleep. I often let him sleep in until eight o'clock. He eats, but without appetite or enjoyment. I do have to admit that the parade of lasagna, frozen dinners, and fast food I'm offering does little to tempt any of us.

He begs me not to make him go to school. *I'm tired*, he com-plains. *My stomach hurts.* So do his arms and legs, his hands, his feet, his little toe, his big toe. I know what is really hurting him, but there is nothing I can do about it. So I give him shot glasses filled with Pepto-Bismol, wrap his leg in ace bandages, fill pans with Epsom salt so he can soak his feet. I treat all the symptoms and have no idea what to do about their underlying cause.

We are constantly late for school. Matthew dawdles over breakfast and complains about whatever clothes I select for him but refuses to select his own. He says it is too cold to go to school, or it's raining too hard. His teacher doesn't like him, he insists, and neither do any of the kids. I know this is not true because I have checked with his teacher. "He seems to do just fine once he's here," his teacher assures me.

We get in the car. "I have to throw up," he says when we are only a few blocks down the street. I dutifully swing over to the side of the road so he can open the door. I'm pretty sure he is faking, but I hate cleaning up vomit and don't want to take any chances. After a few minutes of fake retching, he gives up and closes the door, and we drive on.

We routinely arrive at school long after the buses have left and all the other children are safely tucked away in their classrooms. I plan it this way so that the teachers can't see me dragging this small, damaged child out of the car and across the playground. The other children can't see him as he collapses on me, refusing to go any further until I convince him by threatening to spank his behind.

The school is being renovated, and Matthew's class is housed in a portable building set up at the corner of the playground farthest from the parking lot. I grab an umbrella in one hand and Matthew in the other, and together we trudge through the puddles and around the fenced-in piles of building equipment. To keep his mind off our destination, I keep up a monologue as we walk. "Why, I think that's a cement mixer!" I chirp, or, "My! It looks like they just got a delivery of lumber!" until finally Matthew turns his small, sad face up at me and pleads, "Mom, could you please just not talk?" My forced cheeriness is wearing on my nerves, too.

The Grief Group

chapter twenty-four

In the mail, there's another letter from the Coroner's Office.

This one is smaller and flatter than the autopsy report had been. Inside is a single sheet of letterhead on which is printed an invitation to join a counseling session for "those who have recently experienced the loss of a loved one."

The boys and I are still going to see Adrienne, the family counselor, but I'm ready to call it quits. Matthew still refuses to speak to her; Adrienne tells me that they spent their last two sessions playing board games in silence. Nikolaus is more talkative but is starting to balk at the time commitment. "There are a thousand things that are more helpful than talking to her," he tells me. These thousand helpful things seem to boil down to hanging around with his friends and watching TV, but I'm not inclined to argue with him.

I can't help wondering if there are better things I could

be doing to help my children, to help myself. I call the number listed on the coroner's letter for more information on the counseling session.

"Is the group mostly older women?" I ask.

"We have two groups for people who are experiencing loss," the soothing voice replies. "You can pick the group that feels most comfortable for you. One group is primarily for people over fifty-five. Their concerns tend to be different than those in our younger loss group, which is designed for people in their thirties or forties."

The thought of meeting people my age who have lost spouses is intriguing. Do they have the same issues list that I do? How are they coping? What are they doing to help their kids? Have they been able to communicate with their spouses after death?

One night, I cruise the Internet looking for information on widows, specifically young widows. The results are not encouraging. According to the U.S. Census, in 1995, there were more than thirteen million widows and widowers in the United States. More than ten million of them are over sixty-five. Nationwide, there are fewer than five hundred thousand widows and widowers under the age of forty-five. My chances of finding these people on my own are fairly slim. So far, I haven't met any other widows my age. I decide that the group is my best shot.

I arrive at the counseling center a few minutes before eight o'clock and check in with an elderly receptionist. I show her my letter. "Coping with Grief," she chirps, giving me a big smile as if the letter says I won the lottery. "First door on the left."

The designated room offers a circle of chairs with a box of tissues on every other one and a card table with ice water, coffee, and name tags. Although the session is scheduled to start in two minutes, I'm the only one here. Suppressing the urge to bolt, I take a name tag and a cup of water and sit in one of the chairs facing the door.

A small, blond woman enters the room and hovers uncertainly between the refreshments and the circle. She is young, no more than twenty-five. She could be a volunteer checking the coffee set-up, but I know she is not. There is something in her slow walk, in her wearied expression, that tells me she's one of the group. I am about to say hello when she retreats quickly back out the door.

A man sticks his head through the doorway. "Is this Surviving Divorce?" he asks. I shake my head. "Two doors down on your left," says a large woman with short, gray hair who is entering behind him. This place is a corridor of human misery.

The gray-haired woman fills out a name tag in big, bold strokes and slaps it on her chest. It says MARIE. She is big in a square, stocky way, solid rather than flabby. Her light-blue tracksuit looks a bit too snug to be comfortable, and her hair is uneven, as if she tried to cut it herself.

As Marie pours a cup of coffee, another woman enters, and then a man, and then another man. We acknowledge each other with short nods, and then, just one beat too abruptly, we each look away. I surreptitiously watch the newcomers shuffle around the refreshment table in silence, maintaining a careful distance as they fill in their name tags, take coffee or water, and find a seat. In a few minutes, we are all settled, and then we wait, each in our own space, arms crossed or hands folded around white paper cups, staring at the floor or our laps.

Because I know they will not look up, I can openly study each person without embarrassment. John is a large man with thinning hair, an enormous stomach, and a dirty flannel shirt. His habit of rubbing his hands up and down his upper thighs, as he is doing now, has worn white streaks down the front of his jeans. Kyle is thin and red haired, with leather loafers and knife-like creases in his khaki pants. He holds his Styrofoam cup at arm's length as though he's afraid it might spontaneously spill.

Next to Marie, who is fiddling with the strap of her orthopedic sandal, sits a small, serene woman named Abra. Her olive skin does little to hide the dark circles under her eyes.

I fight the urge to get up and leave.

We wait in silence except for the fluorescent buzz. There are still two empty chairs. A new woman enters the room, and we all look up at her. She has long, gray hair that looks uncombed. She is wearing a flowered skirt that swirls against her legs as she strides to one of the remaining empty seats in the circle. Her name tag is encased in plastic and reads "Sunny." She says, "Good evening, everyone. This group is for those who are coping with grief. Before we begin, I just want to make sure you are all where you expect to be." She makes deliberate eye contact with each of us in turn.

I want to say that I'm really not where I expected to be at all, but I keep quiet. Sunny continues in a soft, slow voice. "We are all here because we are experiencing the loss of someone close to us. Marie and Kyle have been here before." Everyone looks at Marie and Kyle. "For the rest of you who are new, let me tell you what to expect."

Sunny tells us that she is not a therapist but a trained volunteer. She emphasizes the training. She tells us that her husband died of cancer many years ago. Her children were small then; they are grown now. She's been a group leader for four years. "Believe me, I still remember what it felt like to sit where you are sitting and feel the pain that you are all feeling now. I'm glad that you all decided to come and share that pain with each other."

Then Sunny switches gears and seems to get down to business. "We are here to provide each other with a supportive environment. Try not to ask questions, but instead, make positive comments whenever possible. And refrain from giving each other advice. Instead, try to validate the other person's feelings."

The young blond who had darted away earlier is hovering in the doorway. Sunny motions to her to come in. All eyes move briefly in her direction before returning to focus on coffee cups, shoes, or floor. The blond girl reddens and slips quickly into the last remaining seat, which is next to Sunny.

"Welcome," Sunny says to her. "We are just beginning to introduce ourselves, so you are right on time." The blond looks like she wants to sink into the floor. There is a moment when I think that Sunny will say to her, "So, why don't you start?" But, mercifully, she calls on Marie instead.

Marie takes a deep breath. She says, "I've buried three husbands. My first was killed in Vietnam. I married him when I was sixteen, and we weren't married more than a week when he was sent away. He never came back. I was twenty when I married my second husband. He was a drunk, a mean drunk. I don't think there was anyone who was sad when he died, even his own family. Then I married Charlie. He was the best of the bunch by far. We were both thirty when we got married, and we were married for almost ten years. He's been gone now over two years. My life ain't worth a nickel without him. That's why I come here, almost two years now."

I do the math and figure that Marie is actually younger than I am, but she looks like she's seen some hard years. It horrifies me that Marie has been in this group for two years. Where will I be two years from now? I hope to God I'm not still here.

John is sitting next to Marie. He speaks softly in a slow drawl, rubbing his nicotine-stained fingers on the legs of his worn-through jeans as he speaks. "My partner—I guess that's what I call him—oh, hell, he's just Ben to me, and y'all can call him Ben, too. Ben and I were together for almost twenty years. When we first met, back in 1979, people like us still had to hide.

Ben was older than me by about ten years, but we were what you'd call soul mates. So we moved out here away from our families, and we had each other. That was enough.

"Anyways, about six months ago, he was standing in the kitchen, and all of a sudden he said he was dizzy. Then he keeled over, right into the dog's dish." He shakes his head. His eyes glisten, and he swallows hard. "I was so scared. I drove him over to the hospital, and they had him in that intensive care with needles and tubes and all. I thought he'd be okay."

Tears are tracing tracks down his red cheeks, but he continues, "Well, he lasted three days in there. When he died, they called his sister from Ohio. She hadn't seen Ben in thirty years, but they said I was nothing legal to Ben, so they had to call her. The first thing his sister did was throw me out of the house. Then she made all the funeral arrangements. Never asked me a thing. Never even talked to me. I had to call the church myself to find out when the services were. Anyway, I guess I'm getting off track, but that's why I'm here. Because Ben died, and I miss him terrible."

As John talked, several of us grabbed tissues from the boxes that had been set on the floor when people sat down. Sunny waits until the boxes have been passed around the circle and then turns to the fragile blond. "You don't have a name tag," Sunny says, "but why don't you tell us your name and why you are here?"

The blond begins slowly, shyly, her voice shaking. "My name is Peg. My husband, Butch, died three weeks ago today. Butch was diagnosed with throat cancer about a year ago. We thought he could beat it, but it beat him first."

She details the various treatments, the clinics, the doctors. She speaks in a low, flat voice, not looking at anyone, addressing some middle distance. "The doctors finally said there was nothing more they could do, so I brought Butch home," she says. "He only lived a few weeks after that, but at least he was home."

The Grief Group

It hits me suddenly that none of the stories I will hear tonight are going to have happy endings. No one will say, "And then he went through chemo, and he's been in remission ever since." Or, "The lesions went away, and it turned out to be nothing." Or, "Then the car swerved just in time and missed hitting the brick wall." A happy ending doesn't lead you to this room. Whatever the beginning, each of our stories has a guaranteed bad ending.

There are two more stories with unhappy endings before it is my turn. I tell the basics of my story quickly. I'm surprised that my voice and hands are shaking, but I don't cry. I'm glad that I don't cry. I look around at the faces in the circle as I speak and realize that they are doing what I had done while they were speaking. Listening, yes, but also evaluating and comparing. *At least I wasn't left with children to take care of,* I see them thinking while I tell my story, just as while hearing their stories, I thought, *At least I wasn't left alone.*

By the time we get all the way around the circle, two hours have passed, and the session is over. I get in my car, open the sunroof, and crank up the stereo. I feel the cool air rush through my hair and the bass line pound against my chest as I drive too fast, grateful to be going back home.

I go to the group two more times before I decide that it's really not much help to me. None of the people in the group seem to have the same concerns as I do. Their lives are too different, their experiences too dissimilar, their concerns too foreign to me. But before the end of the last group I attend, I decide to ask them one final question: "Have any of you had a visit from your spouses since they died?"

John shakes his head. "I sure would like to, though. I wish Ben would come back and tell his sister that it's not right what she's doing."

Marie says, "You know, sometimes, after a few beers, I get the feeling like Bill is sitting beside me. Not Charlie, the one I'm here for. But my second husband, Bill, the drunk. Isn't that something? I'm drinking because of Charlie, but it's Bill sitting there."

I turn to Sunny. "Have any members of your groups ever said they received a sign from their loved ones?"

"Well, truthfully, this is the first time this subject has ever come up," she says.

"I've been thinking a lot about the afterlife," John says, "and I think there is none. I think the reason that Ben hasn't contacted me is that he is just gone, truly gone."

"I like to think that Charlie is somewhere waiting for me," Marie says. "Someplace nice and clean, no drinking allowed. And I hope Bill is resting in hell."

Peg jumps in, "Why should we be so self-important as to think that we are the only living things that go on? Do animals that die in the forest live on in some alternate forest somewhere? Do all the fish live on in some eternal ocean? Does every blade of grass that dies go to some field of grass in the sky, where it is always sunny and they live happily ever after?"

"It's a mystery," Sunny says, impatient to wrap up the discussion. "We can't know it all while we are still alive. We only get divine wisdom after death."

"Maybe we don't get divine wisdom at all," John responds.

"Maybe when you die, you are finally allowed to just give up," Marie says. "You can just let go and die."

"Maybe that's all there is," Peg says slowly, "but I want more. I would give anything to see Butch again, to feel his presence somehow. But more and more now, I don't think that it's going to happen."

As much as I hate to admit it, I don't think it's going to happen, either.

Other Ways to Cope

chapter twenty-five

"I don't know why you'd want to hang around with a group of people who are more depressed than you are," Annemarie says, stubbing out the third cigarette she's finished in the hour I've been in her kitchen. The occasional cigarette that was helping her cope with her divorce has quickly turned into a full-blown habit. "What you need is to go out and have some fun."

The word "fun" sounds like it comes from another language, a language I knew once but have since forgotten. "I don't know what fun means," I say. I realize that I'm wallowing in self-pity, but for the moment, I don't care. "Fun doesn't apply to me anymore."

Annemarie leans over and pulls a small, brown bottle off the counter and pushes it across the table toward me. "You need to ask you doctor for some of these," she says.

I study the label. It says, "Take one tablet a day, at bedtime."

"It's an antidepressant," Annemarie says, shaking a fresh

cigarette out of a half-empty pack. "It will help you relax. It will help you remember what fun feels like."

I put the bottle back on the table and push it firmly back toward her. "I can't take any drugs."

"Your doctor will prescribe them for you if you ask," Annemarie says. "Everyone takes them."

"I can't take drugs. I have to stay alert. I have to be able to drive."

"You can still drive when you take these. They just make you feel better–happier."

"Do they help you sleep?" I ask. I honestly can't remember having slept at all in the two months since Nick died. I lie in bed for hours each night, waiting for sleep, waiting for Nick. I must doze off at some point, but I don't remember waking up. Sleeping and eating are just things I go through the motions of doing.

"They don't make you sleepy, but you'll feel calmer, so you'll probably be able to sleep better. Mainly, you'll feel more positive. You'll smile more." She demonstrates by flashing me a big smile.

I'm not sure I want to be happier. What would Nikolaus and Matthew think if suddenly I went around smiling all the time? Still, a drug-induced sleep sounds enticing, like an escape that might do wonders. But what if something happened while I was sleeping? What if Matthew cried out or Nikolaus was suddenly sick and needed me? What if I couldn't wake up?

Taking anything, even a glass of wine, just seems like too big a risk. Anyway, it seems unfair to the kids to start drinking or taking medication. Their loss is at least as great as mine, maybe greater, and nobody is suggesting that they start drinking or that I feed them "happy pills." It takes very little alcohol to knock me out. I don't want to worry about the kids coming home from school and finding me passed out on the couch. I don't want to turn into one of those people who can't get out of bed without a pill. I have to stay alert. I have to be ready for anything.

"Thanks, anyway," I say to Annemarie. "I just don't think that it's for me."

—⚙—

It's a rainy day, and Barb and I have taken Matthew and Kevin to the bowling alley. Matthew seems to be enjoying throwing the ball as hard as he can down the lane.

"What about that counselor you were going to?" Barb asks. "I thought going to counseling as a family was a good idea."

"I did, too," I say, "but Matthew won't talk to her at all. So I told her that I wouldn't force him to go anymore. The counselor actually agreed with me."

"You have to get Matthew to talk," Barb says. "He just doesn't seem to be himself since Nick died. Did you talk to the psychologist at his school?"

"I did. She told me she specializes in learning disabilities and doesn't have the time or training to deal with Matthew. She gave me a number for a counseling service."

"Did you call?"

I nod. "It was a suicide hotline." Kevin throws a strike, and the video monitor hanging above the lane plays a cartoon in which a cannonball blasts away a set of bowling pins. Matthew watches it intently, smiling.

—⚙—

I have an appointment with my doctor to get my eye checked. I had called my doctor a few days after the injury, and he had prescribed some drops to help it heal. The drops are all gone now, and my eye seems to be okay, but I don't want to take any chances.

"You've lost weight," my doctor comments as he examines my eye. "Are you still in pain?"

"No, my eye feels fine."

"Are you sleeping?" he asks, sounding concerned. I know he's thinking about Nick's death now, not my eye.

"No. At least, I don't think I am."

"Would you like a prescription to help you sleep? I could also give you an antidepressant that would help with your appetite."

I shake my head. "I really don't want to take a prescription. I don't want to be drugged."

He taps his pen on my chart softly, thinking. "I understand your concern. There are probably too many people who take prescriptions when they don't need to. But you've been through a trauma. There is nothing wrong with taking something to help you get through it."

It is well documented that Jackie took a variety of drugs, both before and after her husband died. "Vitamin" shots to give her energy. Pills to help her sleep. But she had a staff to drive her around. She had nannies to take care of her children.

"I just don't want to take drugs."

"Well, then, maybe just consider Benadryl to help you sleep. It's a mild decongestant, but it also makes you drowsy. It won't knock you out, and it's not addictive."

That night, I take two Benadryl before going to bed. It fails to make me drowsy. Again, I lie awake, staring at the ceiling, my mouth so dry it aches.

The Letter

chapter twenty-six

M any weeks pass before I find the letter.

I find it in the middle of the night. I am sleepless, restless, so I sit in my office, shuffling papers but not accomplishing much. Nick's briefcase is next to my desk, and I decide that emptying it is something I can get done.

Inside I find business cards, a handful of pens, a granola bar, a flashlight with extra batteries. Just like Nick to be prepared for anything. I pull out an electronic date book. When I flip it on, it demands a password. I try a few obvious ones—his birthday, my birthday, our wedding anniversary, various nicknames—with no success. I put the date book aside.

His briefcase has several pockets. I run my hand through each one to assure they are empty. This nets me a package of tissues, a flat, brown paper bag, and a small, white envelope.

Inside the paper bag are four valentines and a receipt. One

valentine has a bunny surrounded by hearts—for Matthew, no doubt. Another contains the kind of crude bathroom humor that Nikolaus loves. One of the two remaining cards has large hearts and flowers on the front and a poem inside, and the other has a mildly suggestive cartoon on the front. I remember all the times Nick slipped valentines under my pillow, on my dashboard, even once in the refrigerator—any unexpected place. I remember the last dozen roses he sent, the ones that he specially ordered in advance, the ones that arrived a week after he died, their dried petals now resting in a crystal dish on my dresser. I think again how lucky I am to have had such an extraordinary marriage, such a wonderful husband.

I put the valentines back in the bag and turn my attention to the small, white envelope. It reads "Nick" in swirling loops of blue ink, and the flap is open. The card inside has a picture of a sailboat on it. There is no preprinted message, only a handwritten note:

Friday, Feb. 6
My dearest Nick—

I want to thank you for being so gentle last night, but then that is the way you always are. I need you so much. I am glad that you were there for me.

You mean more to me than you can ever know. I hope that someday we can be together.

—Kathy

A blackness begins to form around the edges of the words, closing in around them. The note falls from my hands, but the words still sting my eyes. *"so gentle tonight . . . I need you . . . we can be together . . . "* Another woman. Kathy. An office romance. An affair.

I feel a deep vibration shake my body, and it takes me a

moment to realize that it is because there is a long, low moan coming from my own throat. I clap my hands over my mouth to silence myself. *The children,* I think. *Must not wake the boys.*

I am cold, shaking. The note lies on the floor where I dropped it. I circle it cautiously as if it might make a sudden move. Then, I pick it up and stuff it back into the envelope. Should I destroy it? No. Hide it. Yes, hide it.

I thrust the envelope into the pocket of my robe, relieved to have it out of sight but afraid to lose track of it. I go down to the living room. Nick's picture rests on the mantel. "How could you?" I hiss. He smiles back, oblivious. I want to smash his picture. I want to throw it against the wall. I want to stomp on his stupid smile. But the boys are sleeping. How could I explain why I took their father's picture and smashed it, threw it against the wall, stomped on it? I must remain in control. Sleep is out of the question. I can't even sit down. I pass the endless night pacing, trying to figure out what to do next.

At seven, I wake the boys. I make them breakfast and help them organize their books, lunches, and jackets. It's a normal morning, yet everything has changed. I put on jeans and a sweatshirt and drive Matthew to school, the small, square envelope jabbing at my leg from inside my jeans pocket. I return to the empty house and close the door behind me. Only then do I let go—with sobbing, screaming cries that tear my throat and make my head pound. I'm choking, I'm drowning. I can't catch my breath. I shriek through the empty rooms. "You bastard! Where are you?" I want to talk to him right now.

Later, calmer, I decide I must know the truth. I must find out. I pick up the phone and call the switchboard at Nick's office. In a moment, Kathy is on the phone.

"I'm Nick Lenhart's wife," I begin. "You may remember me."

"Of course, Gloria," Kathy says, and then waits for me to continue.

"I'm calling because I found a note that you wrote to my husband. I'm wondering what it was about."

She is unruffled. "It was just a thank you note. He was very kind to me one night when I was having some personal problems. He was a very caring man, very gentle and sweet, very sensitive—"

I cut her off. "I know what he was like. I was married to him for ten years. What was your relationship with him?"

I want her to assure me that they were no more than business associates, perhaps even good friends. I want her to tell me that I'm misinterpreting her note, reading it all wrong, jumping to conclusions. But instead she says, "Nick and I had a very special relationship. I understood him at a deeper level than most people. He was always there for me when I needed help with a business or personal problem. We went through so much together."

In my fury, I cut to the chase. "So, did you fuck him?"

She gives a satisfied chuckle. "No, we hadn't gotten that far yet. I think we both knew it was inevitable, but of course I understood that he had obligations to deal with. . . ."

She would have gone on, but I had heard more than enough. "You are sick," I say and slam down the phone.

Just before noon, the doorbell rings. I ignore it. It rings again. I hear Janine's voice calling, "Gloria, are you in there?"

I open the door and she says, "I thought we were going out to lunch today." She sees my rumpled clothes, uncombed hair, tear-streaked face. "But it looks like you're having a bad day."

"No. No," I say. "Perfect day. I'll just get ready." I have to pull myself together.

"You've been holding everything in for too long," Janine

says, arm around my shoulder, leading me toward the couch. "You have every right to be sad. It's better to just let it go."

I try to speak, to explain that this about more than Nick's death, but my words come out in gulps. Finally, I take the envelope out of my pocket and hand it to her. She looks at the rumpled square, confused. "Read it," I say, and she does.

"Who is she?" Janine asks.

"She worked with Nick."

"Have I met her? Was she at the funeral?"

"She was wearing the hat."

"Oh my God, I remember her."

"She says she didn't fuck him," I say.

"When did she say that?" Janine asks.

"When I called her."

"You called her?" Janine's eyes widen in disbelief.

I nod. "She told me how wonderful Nick was. I said, 'I know, I've been married to him for ten years.'"

"Did you ask her if she fucked him?"

"How else would I have found out?"

"What did she say?"

"She said no—not yet."

Janine looks relieved. "Well, that's it then. They didn't fuck."

"But she said they were going to. They hadn't yet only because Nick 'had obligations.' Obligations like me and the kids."

"Only a bitch would wear a hat like that." Janine puts the letter down. "What are you going to do?"

"What *can* I do? It's not like I can leave him."

Janine looks perplexed. We sit on either end of the couch with the note on the empty cushion between us. Nick continues to smile down from the mantel.

The doorbell rings, and Janine goes to the door.

Annemarie's voice drifts up from the foyer, followed by Janine's hushed tones. She must have brought Annemarie up to speed because when they come into the living room together, Annemarie picks up the note and, without a word, sits down to read it. I don't have the energy to stop her.

"Do you know this woman?" Annemarie asks.

"Not well. She worked with Nick."

"What does she look like?"

Janine answers her. "She was the blond at the funeral in the hat and the three-inch fuck-me heels."

"Is she single?"

"No, I'm pretty sure she's married. In fact, I think she's been married more than once."

"That figures," Janine says, then looks embarrassed as she remembers Annemarie's divorce. "She's just young and stupid."

"Actually, she's about my age," I say. "She just dresses like she's young."

"She dresses like a whore," Janine says.

Annemarie nods. "The note was written the Friday before Nick died. So this little liaison happened on Thursday. Do you remember where he said he was that night?"

I think for a moment. "Scouts meetings are on Thursdays. That Thursday, he called around dinnertime and said he'd be late. He was home by the time we got back from Scouts, though."

"So he didn't spend the night with her." Annemarie is thoughtful. "You know, Hat Woman just doesn't seem like Nick's type."

"A woman like that is every man's type," I retort. "Anyway, the proof is in your hands."

Annemarie waves the letter dismissively. "I'm not so sure. Do you have any other clues?"

"No, unfortunately I've been fairly clueless up till now."

"That's exactly my point. When your husband is having an affair, you usually suspect."

"Hat Woman says she didn't sleep with him," Janine adds.

"When did she say that?" Annemarie looks startled.

"When I called her," I reply feebly.

Annemarie practically jumps out of her chair. "You called her?"

"Yes, I called her." I am suddenly bone tired.

"What did you say?"

I review the highlights of the conversation again, and then, suddenly, I remember something. "I found Valentine's Day cards in his briefcase. I thought they were both for me, but maybe one of them was for her."

Annemarie stops pacing. "Let me see them."

I go upstairs and retrieve the bag. Janine and Annemarie examine the valentines. "Which one do you think was for her?" Janine asks.

"Neither one," Annemarie says. "This receipt says he bought these Valentines at lunchtime on Thursday. I can't picture Nick buying valentines for you, his mistress, and the kids all in one trip. Nick didn't strike me as the Jack Kennedy type, juggling multiple mistresses and a family at the same time."

Janine sighs. "Poor Jackie. Think of what she had to put up with."

This is the last straw. "I've had it with Jackie!" I shriek. "What is so great about Jackie? She had nannies. She had financial advisors. She had teams of lawyers. She took drugs."

Annemarie and Janine are speechless. There is a long moment of silence, then Annemarie says softly, "Jackie had a husband who cheated on her. You didn't."

Janine's face brightens. "Didn't he send you flowers for Valentine's Day?"

I'm not convinced. "It was probably a standing order."

"And when he decided to have an affair, he just forgot to cancel it? I doubt it. But let's call the florist and find out." Annemarie marches over to the desk and picks up the phone.

I'm horrified. "Don't call the florist. I don't want anyone to know that I suspect Nick of having an affair. I'm sorry I even told you two."

"Don't worry, we won't tell a soul. I'll tell the florist that I'm your accountant and I'm calling to verify the bill."

I leave them to use the phone in the living room, and I go into the kitchen to make a cup of tea. I can't bear to listen. In a few minutes, Annemarie and Janine come down the stairs, smiling.

"The florist said that Nick called himself on January 31," Janine says. "He ordered two sets of flowers: one for you and a smaller arrangement for his mother." Elisabeth's arrangement was on her doorstep when I took her home that day. I hid the card and told her that I sent it from the boys.

I'm not ready to be convinced. "Maybe he ordered *hers* from a different florist."

Annemarie rolls her eyes. "You are missing the point. A man who is having an affair does not make sure that his wife has roses on Valentine's Day by placing the order two weeks in advance."

"So what are you saying? I'm imagining the affair? I'm imagining the note?"

"What you are missing is that Hat Woman may be a bunny boiler," Janine says.

"A what?"

"A bunny boiler," Janine repeats. "You remember that movie *Fatal Attraction*? Glenn Close and Michael Douglas have a fling, but then he tries to blow her off because he's really in love with his wife. But Glenn Close won't let it go."

"Yeah, and then Glenn Close breaks into his house and puts his kids' rabbit in a pot of boiling water," Annemarie continues.

"Exactly," Janine adds, satisfied.

"Is this story supposed to be making me feel better?" I ask.

"The point is," Janine says, "that Michael Douglas wasn't in love with Glenn Close at all, it was just a fling. Only Glenn Close wanted it to be something more."

"Right," Annemarie says. "Hat Woman is probably making more of this than it ever really was. She even admits that there was no real affair. The whole thing is probably all in her mind."

"Unfortunately, the only person who could absolutely confirm that for you," Janine says, gesturing toward Nick's picture, "is not able to."

After Janine and Annemarie leave, I drive to the video store and try to rent *Fatal Attraction*, but the only copy is checked out. I'm not sure I need to see it again, anyway. I vividly remember Glenn Close slinking around Michael Douglas's house, stalking his wife, and spying on his children. Up until now, I hadn't noticed anyone unusual slinking around the house or the kids, but then, neither did Michael Douglas's wife in the movie.

I arrive at Matthew's school thirty minutes earlier than usual. I park on one side of the schoolyard and wait, watching for anything unusual, any people who seem like they don't belong there.

When Matthew is safely in the car, I swing by the high school, hoping to spot Nikolaus. I find him talking with a crowd of friends. "Want a ride home?" I call out the window.

"We're all going to Taco Bell to get something to eat," he calls back.

"How about if I give you all a ride?"

"Thanks anyway, but it's only a couple of blocks."

"Don't talk to any strangers," I warn.

"I won't," he responds sarcastically. "Even if they offer me candy."

The crying has exhausted me, even more than usual, and to-night, I know there is no point in staying awake, waiting for Nick to show up. He'd probably be afraid to show his face to me right now anyway.

For the first time in months, I go to bed early, and I sleep all the way through till dawn.

Therapy

chapter twenty-seven

Nick and I went to see a marriage counselor last year. After almost ten years of marriage, we had the usual complaints: Nick was spending too much time at work, I was too involved with the kids, our lives were too stressful, we weren't communicating all that well. Nick's friend Glenn and his wife, Julie, had been to see a counselor and said it was the best thing that ever happened to them. "It's really helped us communicate on a deeper level," Julie told me. Nick thought counseling was a waste of time and money, and he went under protest, only because I insisted. We went once a week for about six months before we agreed that our time and money would be better spent on a weekly night out.

Our therapist, Ryan, has an office in a large, shabby house on a busy street in Berkeley. The sexual ambiguity of the therapist's name seemed to assure us that she wouldn't take sides. Each time we'd visit, I'd have to push the overgrown shrubbery aside in order to climb the broken cement steps that angled sharply up from the street.

"This place needs a paint job," I said to Nick in a conciliatory whisper the first time we stood in front of the smudged glass door.

"This place needs a bulldozer," he grumbled back.

The lower lobby was gloomy and dank with a smell that reminded me of the innumerable houses my mother dragged me to as a child to visit some elderly lady she had met in church or through her bridge group. If Ryan had been dressed in Indian prints and sandals—as I half expected, this being Berkeley—Nick would not have lasted past the first meeting. But she turned out to be a tiny, straightforward woman with neatly cropped, gray hair who dressed casually in linen slacks and a cotton sweater. We scheduled a standing Saturday-morning appointment, although in the beginning, there were several times when Nick and I had separate meetings. Now, I wonder if Nick told Ryan about Kathy. And I wonder if Ryan would tell me.

"I haven't seen you in a long time," Ryan says as I seat myself on her couch and she settles into a facing armchair. "I was wondering how you were doing." She had phoned me weeks ago when she first heard that Nick died; I had assured her that everything was fine.

"I was doing pretty well until yesterday, when I found this." I take the letter out of my purse and pass it to her. She puts on half-glasses and reads it slowly, expressionless, and then pauses thoughtfully and reads it again. Finally, she lowers the paper and asks in her cool, professional tone, "What do you think about this?"

"I came here to ask you that."

"Do you know anything about this woman?"

"Not really. She worked with Nick. She is married—in fact, I think she's been married a few times."

"That doesn't sound like someone Nick would be attracted to. Nick seemed to value loyalty and consistency."

"Those are not the qualities this woman mentioned when I called and asked her about the letter."

"You called her?" Ryan's eyes widen behind her glasses.

Why is everyone surprised by this? I wonder. "Yes, I called her. I asked her to explain this letter."

"What did she say?"

I tell her about my conversation with Kathy. I tell her that Kathy told me that she and Nick didn't sleep together because Nick had "obligations." "She could have been lying about that, though," I say.

"What would motivate her to lie? She clearly didn't care about sparing your feelings. It would be more likely for her to lie and tell you they had slept together."

I'm paying Ryan for this hour, so I decide to get right to the point. "Do you think Nick was having an affair?" I ask. "Did he tell you that he was thinking about leaving me for this woman?"

A look of surprise crosses Ryan's face so quickly, I almost miss it; then she falls back into her familiar noncommittal therapist expression. "I thought Nick seemed focused on improving his marriage, not destroying it."

I thought so too, and I am happy to hear Ryan confirm it. But I still need more reassurance. "But he was also human," I argue. "If she didn't mean anything to him, why did he keep the letter? Why didn't he just throw it away?" I had had time to think up a million questions and was hoping Ryan could help me see the answers.

Ryan thinks for a moment. "The most obvious answer is that he didn't have time to dispose of it. He received it the day before he died. You could argue that he kept it because it's flattering, a boost for his ego. But it's just as likely that he was planning to confront this woman with it on Monday. She worked for him, so my guess is that he would have to deal with this matter directly in some way."

I hadn't thought of this line of reasoning, but it made sense. Kathy worked *for* Nick. Fooling around with her would have jeopardized Nick's job. Would he jeopardize his marriage? Maybe. Would he jeopardize his job *and* his marriage? Nick wouldn't do that, not in a million years. I take the first deep breath I've taken since I found the letter and let it out slowly, feeling the tension drain from my neck and shoulders, feeling my jaw unclench.

Ryan is rereading the letter. She asks, "Besides this letter, do you have any other reason to believe Nick was having an affair?"

"Not really." Suddenly I'm tense again. What did I miss? I've been through his closet and his car. I've searched all his pockets and picked through his credit card receipts. I haven't found any other love notes or any unexplainable receipts, or gifts, or fancy underwear.

Ryan is thoughtful. "There is something odd about this letter," Ryan says slowly. "It just seems very one-sided. She uses phrases like 'I need,' 'I want,' 'I hope.' It doesn't seem to reflect a mature love relationship. It sounds more like a juvenile infatuation, a fantasy."

Like a bunny boiler. Fear is back again in full force. "Do you think I should be worried about this woman stalking me or the kids?" I ask.

"I don't think so," Ryan says, looking at me with a bit more concern than before. "After all, what this woman really wanted was Nick. And he's no longer available. My guess is that she's already moved on to someone else."

Losing It

chapter twenty-eight

Leaving Ryan's, I decide to pay a visit to the cemetery. I don't know what satisfaction I expect to get there. The visit to Ryan's had clarified things for me. Maybe Nick didn't do anything wrong. Maybe it's true that this woman is just a stalker. But I am still angry. This would be an excellent time for Nick to come back and reassure me. Going to visit his grave is the closest to him I'm going to get.

Elisabeth and I were just at the cemetery three days ago. We have gotten in the habit of going about once a week. Nick's grave is still marked by the glass vase with artificial flowers that I planted in the ground where his headstone will eventually go. I look over at Dominick's headstone, polished and shiny as always. *I bet you never betrayed* your *wife,* I think.

Each week, Elisabeth and I bring new flowers out to decorate the grave. I've given up on fresh flowers; the deer eat them.

But artificial flowers disappear almost as fast. Elisabeth says they are stolen by people who come to visit their loved ones and forget to bring their own. Once, after a particularly nice arrangement went missing, I spent an hour searching for the grave that it had been moved to, but I gave up before I found it. Elisabeth says she will show me how to prevent these thefts by tying the flowers to the headstone—once Nick *has* a headstone, she reminds me. People who forget flowers don't bring scissors, she says, and indeed, the flowers she ties to Nick's father's headstone never disappear.

The grass over Nick's grave has not grown in well, so if I see the groundskeeper around, I will ask him to reseed it. In the first few weeks, there were several times when long, deep crevices appeared in the grave, which the groundskeeper told me is normal for fresh graves. "We don't like to push down too much when we bury the caskets," he told me. "They settle in by themselves after the first couple of rains."

Now, however, I am so mad at Nick that I don't care if the earth has sunken in on top of him. I don't care if he has no grass, if his grave is a muddy pit. I don't care if his flowers get stolen.

As I approach, I see that the flowers Elisabeth and I brought three days ago are still there. But there is something else there, too. Lying on the soft, brown earth in front of my vase is a bouquet of artificial lilies tied with a white ribbon.

I believe I know who the flowers are from, but I try to think of any other possibilities. Elisabeth has just been here with me; she doesn't drive, and it's unlikely she would have asked a neighbor to take her again so soon. I can't think of anyone else who would have left such a big, expensive bouquet. It had to be Hat Woman. Ryan was right. She wouldn't waste her time going after me or the children. She's only interested in Nick. She'll be haunting his grave forever, like Joe DiMaggio leaving a rose on Marilyn Monroe's grave every year. I'll never be rid of her.

Losing It

I pick up the lilies and throw them as far away as I can. Lilies are not very aerodynamic; they land only about ten feet away. I walk over and kick them as hard as I can, which only drives them back another few yards. I feel my anger rising. "Get away, you bitch," I scream, kicking at the flowers, stamping on them, smashing them into the mud. The ribbon comes undone, and the bent and soiled flowers are scattered over a small radius. I give each one a last kick and then turn and stomp back to the car. I feel a lot better.

That night, I get a call from Tina. "I went to Nick's grave yesterday," she says, "and I left some flowers. It's really so peaceful there. . . ."

Navigating the
Bureaucracy

chapter twenty-nine

After my meeting with Darla at Mervyn's, the thrill of expecting to receive a lump sum of money that will solve my problems is short-lived. It is quickly overtaken by the reality that getting access to the money will not be easy. And the actual amount I will wind up with turns out to be less than anticipated.

About a month after my meeting with Darla, a check arrives from Mervyn's, along with a letter indicating that it constitutes a payout of the salary Nick had put aside to be paid after retirement. Despite the fact that the letter states that these funds must be paid in full upon death, the enclosed check is a little more than half of the amount that Darla had listed for deferred salary. I call Darla.

"We are required to withhold taxes," she explains. "Check with your tax advisor. You may be able to get some of that back."

"I doubt that you'll get any back," our tax guy says when I explain the situation. "In fact, you may owe even more. The IRS looks at that check as income, which will probably push you into a higher tax bracket." I put the check in the bank and use some of it to pay off the utilities and the phone bill, and then I make small payments on each credit card.

Darla sends me paperwork to convert Nick's retirement accounts. The paperwork warns that there are substantial penalties if I withdraw these funds before I am fifty-five—which is more than ten years from now. Having already lost almost half of one check to taxes, I can't risk even more substantial penalties. I sign the paperwork to convert the accounts to my name, but that does nothing to help my immediate financial problems.

I am named as beneficiary on Nick's retirement account with Mervyn's, so it is easy to transfer it over to my name. But then, when I was looking through our financial files searching for signs of infidelity, I found a spreadsheet on which Nick had listed all the bank and investment accounts we had, along with contact names and numbers. According to this spreadsheet, Nick had two 401(k) accounts from previous employers, which he had invested with a mutual fund company. I need those accounts transferred into my name, too, but that's not going to be so simple.

I call the first contact number on the spreadsheet. By the time I get to speak with a live person at this company, I'm already braced for trouble. I have yet to encounter the option that tells me, "Press four if your husband is dead and you want to retrieve your money," so I usually just press zero repeatedly until a live person comes on the line. But in this case, my usual tactic does not work and I'm forced to listen to four different menus before I'm allowed to speak with a human.

When I explain my situation to the company representative I'm finally transferred to, he tells me to send a death certificate.

"A death certificate is no problem," I say, relieved. Everyone

I talk to wants a death certificate. Death certificates cost four dollars each, and I have already used fifteen of them by filing claims for life insurance and Social Security and to get access to bank balances and brokerage accounts. They're expensive but easy to get.

"We also need an affidavit of domicile," he continues, bored, "and it must be notarized."

I'm familiar with this form, too. An affidavit of domicile is a two-page legal form, and if you read through all the wherefores and wherebys, it says that Nick was a resident of California when he died. I know this because the adoption lawyer, Jerry, referred me to one of the estate lawyers in his office, who charged me six hundred dollars to produce this and several other forms that were required to retrieve about one thousand dollars from one of Nick's speculative brokerage accounts.

It was a good investment, though. I now have a file of six different legal documents that I can pull out when someone asks for them. I simply pull the necessary form out of my file, photocopy it, and go downtown to pay the guy at One-Hour Instant Photo ten dollars to notarize my signature. The guy at One-Hour Instant Photo has tattoos and a nose ring, but a supervisor at my bank told me that he's the only one in town who provides notary services. One-Hour Instant Photo Guy seems to take this responsibility very seriously. Although I find myself in his shop two or three times a week for notary services, each and every time, he carefully studies my driver's license photo and then matches it carefully to my face.

The mutual fund guy I have on the phone sounds like he's shuffling through papers. "What did you say your name is?" he asks. When I tell him, he says, "Then you are not the named beneficiary."

"Who is the named beneficiary?" I ask. This is going to be like pulling teeth.

"Rachael Lenhart."

"Oh, that was my husband's first wife," I say. "She's dead."

"I'll connect you to a supervisor," he says, and I hear a click.

After ten minutes on hold, the supervisor comes on. She's no more lively than the first guy. "We need a death certificate and a notarized affidavit of domicile for each of the deceased," she says, "and a marriage certificate, a certified copy of the will, and Letters Testamentary."

I ask her to repeat the list several times until I have written down all of the required documents. "Once you get these documents, then I can transfer the account?" I ask.

"No, then we will make a determination," she says. Financial institutions are always making determinations. Often they determine that you need to send them more paperwork. Sometimes they simply need additional copies of what you've already sent. Of course, they can't just make the copies themselves. You have to send them more "originals." They see no irony in this request. I've learned it's best to just produce as many originals as they need by trotting off to One-Hour Instant Photo until the institution is finally satisfied and can make the determination to send me my own money.

This time, however, I've got a new problem. One of the items on the list is not in my file: Letters Testamentary. I put in a call to the estate lawyer's paralegal. It only costs eighty dollars an hour to talk with her, versus the one hundred and sixty-five dollars it costs me to speak with my lawyer. "Letters Testamentary are issued by the probate court," his paralegal informs me. "Tell them you don't need them."

I submit the rest of the papers and call the mutual fund company two weeks later to follow up. "Your file seems to be complete," a different representative tells me. "Except for Letters Testamentary, which we have not received."

I explain how Letters Testamentary are only issued by a

probate court. I explain that since I wasn't required to go through probate, I didn't get these documents, and in fact, I don't need them at all. She puts me on hold for ten minutes, and when she returns, she says, "Our staff attorney says Letters Testamentary are necessary to make a determination."

I put in another call to my lawyer's paralegal. "They won't give me my money without Letters Testamentary."

"Tell them that in California, you don't need them," the paralegal says.

"They are in Minnesota," I say, "and they insist on having them." I decide to spring for ten minutes of the lawyer's time and ask to be transferred.

"There is nothing we can do," he says. "They are asking for something that doesn't exist in California. I would advise you to ask to explain that to their counsel directly."

But their counsel is permanently in meetings, or in court, or gone for the day, so I wind up having several more conversations with various representatives. "A determination cannot be made on your file until we receive Letters Testamentary," each one patiently repeats, oblivious to my protests.

I look through the file of legal papers my lawyer has already prepared. I have an idea. I select one that says that I was married to Nick and have two children. After several tests, I run this form through my copier, taped to a banner I printed from my computer reading "Letters Testamentary," which now appears on the top of the form in a matching typeface. I pay One-Hour Instant Photo Guy ten dollars to scrutinize my driver's license and match it to my face. He puts his stamp on the bottom of my phony Letters Testamentary and has me sign his book. I bring the papers to the post office and get a receipt. Four weeks later, I receive a check.

—⚋—

When Nick's life insurance finally pays out, they don't send a check. Instead, they send a checkbook. I look at the opening balance on the account statement for a long time. If I want to, I can take one of these brand-new checks and write a really big number on it, and it will not bounce. If the thought of this did not terrify me, I'd be very happy.

My first impulse is to pay everything off—the credit cards, the mortgage, the car—but I will need some cash to pay for adoption papers, to keep our health insurance current, and to fix the gutter.

I fight the overwhelming urge to throw the checkbook away. I wouldn't have this money if Nick hadn't died. I can't shake the feeling that it is laced with sorrow and guilt. Blood money.

If I had the chance to return the money and get Nick back, get our life back the way it was, I'd do it in a minute. But unfortunately, no one is offering me that option. My only option is to decide how to use the money.

I sort through the bills and pick out the ones that I'd most like to be rid of. I pick out the credit card bills, write a check for each for the full amount, and mark "please cancel" on the part of that statement that I return to the company. Then I pay off the home-equity loan and write checks for three months worth of mortgage payments, and health insurance payments, and car payments. I carefully subtract the amount of each check from the opening balance; when I'm done, I've depleted the account by more than $50,000. I hide the checkbook under some papers in the top desk drawer. In a few days, I hope, I will have forgotten that it's even there.

"I'd buy a house in Hawaii," Karin says, "or take a six-month trip around the world."

"I can't take the kids out of school," I point out.

The waiter comes to bring another pot of tea. Karin is polishing off her green curry, while I'm still pushing my Pad Thai around on my plate.

"Seeing the world would be a better education than they'll get in school," Karin says.

"I'll let you explain that to Ruth Miner. I don't think I'd be allowed to take Nikolaus out of the country while this adoption mess is going on."

"What's happening with the adoption?"

"I've filed the papers requesting appointment as Nikolaus's legal guardian. All of the Miners have received notices from the court, and if they want to object, they have ninety days to request a hearing. If they don't object, I become the legal guardian, and then I can start adoption procedures."

"How is Nikolaus feeling about all this?"

"I'm trying to keep him out of it as much as possible. And he doesn't seem to want to talk about it. He's busy with school, with Scouts, with his friends. And that's where his focus should be, not worrying about adoption issues."

"Do you think the Miners will object to the adoption?"

"I'm not sure. I know that Nikolaus talked to his grandmother about the apartment idea, but I'm not sure where that stands. I guess I'll just have to wait and see if they agree to sign the papers."

At the next table, a young couple is flirting with each other over their hot-and-sour soup. He smiles slyly, she giggles. He is sandy blond, tanned, and very handsome. She is pretty but in a plainer, more wholesome way. He is watching the light dance on her hair. She stares into his eyes when he speaks, her thoughts on something more urgent than whatever he is saying. I remember feeling like they do, being in love like they are. It seems like a long time ago. I wonder if someday someone will tempt him to cheat on her.

"Have you heard anything from Nick?" Karin asks.

"What?"

"Have you made any contact with Nick?" Karin repeats patiently. This is a serious question; she truly believes that the dead can communicate. I want to share this belief, but the more time passes with nothing from Nick, the more hopeless it seems.

"Not a peep. I've begun to think that he doesn't want to talk to me." I haven't told Karin about finding the letter. I haven't told anyone besides Annemarie and Janine, and they are sworn to secrecy. The hurt is too deep, too humiliating, to share.

"Maybe you are not sufficiently open to the communication. If you are doubtful, you can drive the spirit to find a more receptive host."

"I've been open nonstop, twenty-four hours a day, seven days a week, for months. But nothing is getting through." I wonder if Kathy is a receptive host. Maybe while I've been waiting around every night for Nick to show, he's been over communicating with her.

The couple at the next table have asked for the check, and they are now making a game of snatching it out of each other's hands. Finally, he tosses some money on the table, and they walk out hand in hand. Their business suits tell me that they are on their way back to their jobs, back to work. But their smiles, their sideways glances, tell me that he'll be waiting outside her office at five o'clock. Maybe they'll ride the bus together back to her apartment. She'll make him spaghetti, or perhaps they'll go out. Does she know that he will probably die first and she will be left to take care of the kids, the paperwork, his mother? Will she make sure that he lists her as beneficiary on his retirement plan?

"Maybe it's time to get some help." Karin is looking at me with concern.

"I'm already seeing a therapist."

"I don't mean a therapist. I mean someone who can help facilitate communication with Nick."

"Are you still talking about that?" The young couple is gone now and I'm still here with Karin, who thinks it's possible for me to chat with my dead husband, even though she barely spoke to him when he was alive.

"I just think it's time you got someone to help you reach out to Nick."

"Like some sort of psychic? One of those people who predict lottery numbers?" I push my Pad Thai back and try to signal for the waiter's attention.

"I'm not suggesting a TV psychic. But there are people with heightened sensitivities, people who can be very helpful in receiving and interpreting messages."

"If Nick wants to give me a message, why wouldn't he just do it directly?"

"Maybe he's trying and he can't get through. Sometimes it's helpful to have a facilitator, or a translator. Someone who comes from a different perspective can sometimes help you achieve things that you didn't think were possible."

She may have a point. And hadn't Ryan helped me see things in different way? I do want to stay open to the possibility that Nick may be trying to reach me, even though part of me thinks it's outrageous. And I can't help but be wary of someone recognizing my desperate hopes and preying on them.

"Doesn't it cross your mind that these psychics are just charlatans, preying on desperate people?"

"Some are fakes," Karin concedes, "but many are professionals who don't promise to change your life. They can just help you open channels to the other side." The concern in Karin's face is so obviously genuine, it makes me sad. I think, *why not let her help me, if she can.*

"Do you know people like this?"

"I can give you some names if you're interested. But there is one thing I'll warn you about. If you go, you have to go as a believer. Otherwise, you'll just be wasting your time."

That night, as I lie in bed wide awake, I consider her offer. What if Nick is trying to communicate and I just can't hear him? Maybe he's afraid of talking to me now that I know about Kathy. What do I really know about Kathy? Maybe I should give him a chance to explain. Maybe the reason that none of the people in the grief group could communicate with their spouses was that they needed professional help. Karin said I'd have to be a believer. I'm not a believer, but I feel like I could be one—if only I could reach across whatever divides us and be with Nick again. Even if it were only for a moment. Even if I had to go through someone else to do it.

The next morning, I call Karin and ask for a phone number.

Lessons in
Intuition

chapter thirty

I drive cautiously down the narrow street of flat-fronted houses, simultaneously searching for the address and a parking space. The house numbers stop and start over again midway down the block, entirely skipping the one I'm looking for. But I find a parking spot and wedge my car into it on my third try. I hike back up the hill, recounting the house numbers unsuccessfully before finally heading back to my car and my cell phone, cursing myself and my luck.

A cheery voice answers on the first ring. "This is Myah."

"Myah, this is Gloria. I'm lost."

"Where are you?"

"Don't you know? I thought you were a psychic," I say. I know how rude this sounds, but at this point, I don't care. After parallel parking on a forty-five-degree incline and then walking up and down the same block for twenty minutes looking for a nonexistent address, I'm frustrated and annoyed. I'm already sorry I agreed to go through with this—I'm in no mood to communicate with anyone, let alone the dead.

I would like to just turn around and go home, but the voice that comes back to me over the phone is reassuringly normal, even a touch apologetic. I immediately regret being rude.

"Actually I don't claim to be a psychic," she says. "I'm just intuitive. And I'm sensing that you're frustrated."

"You're right about that. I'm on your street, but your house number doesn't seem to exist."

A few clicks and several seconds later, a slim, blond woman holding a cordless phone appears on the porch of the house across the street from my car. She waves, and I trudge across to greet her.

Karin had regaled me with stories of Myah's triumphs: Some friends had been about to buy a house. All the inspections turned out clean, but Myah predicted disaster. They backed out of the deal, and two months later, a heavy rainstorm washed out a major portion of the foundation. Another one of Myah's disciples was choosing between two jobs, one in San Francisco and one out of town. Myah advised her to get out of town. She did, and on the third day of her new job, she met her future husband and lived happily ever after. I still had a healthy dose of skepticism, but at the same time, I needed answers, and I was willing to look for them in unconventional places, so I made the call.

I expect Myah to be old and mystical. Instead, she is a striking blond, about my age, dressed in a black turtleneck and jeans. She welcomes me into a tiny, sunny front room that houses two futons and a collection of Latin American art.

"The house belongs to some people I'm helping," she had explained on the phone when I made the appointment. "Their daughter died of cancer, and I'm helping them sort things out."

She makes herbal tea for us in a tiny kitchen that overlooks an almost vertical backyard. We return to the front room and settle into an overstuffed couch and chair, not much different than the setup I'm used to with Ryan.

She asks me to tell her why I've come. I tell her about Nick. I tell her about our marriage. I tell her about Nikolaus and Matthew. I tell her about my clients, my career. I talk about my life, my dreams, my future, my fears. She turns out to be a very easy person to talk to.

After about forty-five minutes, Myah stops me gently and says, "Now let me meditate on what you have told me." She closes her eyes and lies back against the brightly covered pillows. At first I keep my eyes open, watching her. Then, after a few quiet minutes, with the warm sun streaming through the window and the hot tea settled in my stomach, I suddenly feel very tired. I close my eyes and am just beginning to drift off when Myah speaks.

"You talk about death and despair," she says, "but what I feel around you is a sense of hope. Your aura is at odds with your words. I sense power and direction."

Her eyes are still closed and she falls silent. After a few moments I ask, "Is there more?"

It is another moment before she opens her eyes and continues. "You've had a very bad thing happen to you that you were powerless to control. But you are not out of control. In fact, you have a very strong hold on your inner self. You are steering your life course with a very firm hand."

"But I don't *feel* in control."

"Right now, your energies may be unfocused. When your husband died, you lost a point of reference. An element of your internal navigation disappeared. You feel lost now, but you will only feel this way for a moment. You will soon find a new direction, and your energies will again have focus."

What she says feels true, or at least I'd like to believe it.

I realize that I am no longer thinking of her as a wacko. I ask, "Where will I find this direction?"

Myah smiles. "I don't pretend to see the future. But I feel that you have a powerful force inside you. I know that you will find a way to use it."

I want to ask, *Then what about the house with the screwed-up foundation? What about the woman who took the job and met her husband? How come you could see their futures but not mine?* But I don't. Perhaps it's because I think there is an element of truth in what she is saying. I am a powerful person. I have always believed that I could find my own way. I had come here looking for a peek into the future, but what she is telling me is that it's up to me to shape my own future. Maybe she tells everyone this. But I believe it. I guess I just had to hear someone say it. I had booked a two-hour appointment, but now, halfway through, I am feeling that I've already accomplished a great deal. I haven't communicated with Nick, but I'm feeling better—more powerful and directed—than I have in months.

"Would you like me to read the tarot?" Myah asks.

"Yes, please." As long as I'm here, why not?

"Think about your future," she says as she slowly shuffles the cards. She splays the deck out on the coffee table in front of me and asks me to select four cards. I perform a short charade of carefully selecting some and rejecting others, although actually I feel no special attraction or repulsion toward any of them. They're just cards. She deals a few additional cards in an array around my chosen ones and then studies the display. The center card reads "Justice."

"Yes, I see," she says finally. "There will be some more rocky days ahead, but altogether, the signs are positive." Her eyes are shining, and she raises her head and her voice as if she is addressing a room full of people. "You are in charge and moving forward. You do have a few things blocking your way. But these things will ultimately prove inconsequential, and you will overcome them." *Wow,* I think. *Sign me up.*

"I sense you are concerned about your children," she says. "Do you want to see what the cards say about their future?"

Only if it's good news, I think. But what the heck, I'm on a roll. "Absolutely," I say.

I think about Nikolaus and Matthew as she again shuffles the cards, and again I make a show of selecting a few, pretty much at random. This time, however, the card in the center of the display reveals a skeleton riding a bony horse into a brilliant red sun, with gothic black letters that proclaim DEATH.

"That doesn't look so good," I observe.

"Oh, no, it's very positive," Myah says emphatically.

I am doubtful. This is no longer fun. "Death is positive?"

She nods. "Death is not always interpreted as negative. In this case, it is *very* positive. Death is the primary obstacle that your children will overcome. It will make them stronger." She points to another card. "The King of Cups overflows with good fortune. They will emerge triumphant."

I'm not buying this. The familiar dread is returning, along with the feeling that I should have quit while I was ahead.

"Your older son is a new soul," she says. "You've told me that he is a helper, a healer. The signs of that here are very strong. The cards say that he will take a journey, but it may not mean that he will literally travel. It may also be interpreted as a journey of the mind or the soul.

"Your younger son is an old soul," Myah continues. "I believe he has failed in business in a previous life, a large failure, maybe something on the order of Wall Street in 1929. He is still angry about it, and that anger will drive him. He may feel the need to go back into business. The cards indicate that he will be successful this time."

She must read the incredulity in my face because she says, "I sense that you may not believe everything I say. But believe me, your children have extraordinary inner power. I won't tell you not to worry about them because you're their mother and you will always worry. But I can assure you that they will be okay."

All I can see is the DEATH card staring up at me. It's time to leave. I stand up and fish the envelope of money I got from the ATM this morning out of my purse. I put it on the table, covering the cards. "Thanks, Myah, this has really been great."

She walks behind me to the door. On the steps, I pause. There is one more thing I have to ask.

"Myah, can you feel my husband's presence around me? I'm just wondering. I don't feel him at all, and . . ."

She looks at me sadly, but her voice is firm. "He can't be with you anymore. Spirits only get three days on the earth, and then they have to move on." Of course. I knew that. Three days, three weeks. Whatever. I start down the steps.

"There is one more thing, though," she calls after me, and I stop and turn.

She walks down a few steps to my level. "I get the feeling that your life with your husband was not entirely as you described. I get the feeling that there was some deception. Am I right?"

I say nothing. I had told her a lot about Nick and me, but I purposely hadn't mentioned Hat Woman.

"Don't spend too much time looking back. You can't know what really happened or what might have happened. Just go on with your life, and you'll be fine." She turns, walks back up the stairs slowly, and disappears inside the house.

Losing
the Hat

chapter thirty-one

In the fourteen weeks since Nick died, I've lost a total of twenty-five pounds. Normally, I'd be happy about dropping a few pounds, but the weight loss combined with the lack of sleep has not been a flattering combination. When I look in the mirror, the woman looking back at me is pale and drawn, with large dark circles under her eyes. I live in big baggy sweaters, mostly in shades of black and gray, paired with jeans. It's now mid-May and the weather is starting to get warmer. I think maybe it's time to freshen my look with a few lighter tops and at least one pair of pants that fit. With Nikolaus and Matthew tucked into school for the day, I head to the mall.

The department stores are in full bloom, their floors full of bright pinks, lime greens, pale yellows. Getting off the escalator in my long black coat, I feel like a turd in an Easter basket. I also feel a twinge of guilt. Is it shallow to be shopping for clothes so soon after my husband's death? What if someone I know sees me here, adrift in the cruisewear?

Heading back to my car, I hear a familiar voice call my name. I turn and see Janet, Nick's secretary, crossing the parking lot. "I've been thinking about you a lot," she says, hugging me. "How are you and the boys doing?"

"We are just fine," I lie. "Everything is fine."

Her smile tells me she doesn't believe me. "I want you to know that everyone in the office still feels the loss of Nick," she says. "He definitely left a hole that's going to be hard to fill. It's just not the same without him."

"Thanks so much for saying that," I say sincerely. "It really means a lot to me to know that I'm not the only one who misses him."

"I don't think a day has gone by that I haven't thought about him," Janet says. "It's surprising how deeply his death affected people at work. Do you remember a woman named Kathy? She's been wearing nothing but black since Nick died. I'm actually worried about her. Now she and her husband are going through a divorce." I feel the blood drain from my face, but Janet doesn't notice because she goes on, "And I don't know if you know this, but Rob, who also worked for Nick, has accepted a job with another company. I never thought he would leave Mervyn's, but he said he wants a change."

Janet pauses, suddenly aware that she has said something to upset me. "What I mean is, that losing someone has made us all look at our lives a bit differently than we did before," she says, her face reddening. "I can't even imagine what you are going through."

I put my hand through her arm and give her a reassuring squeeze. "Please tell everyone that the boys and I are fine," I say. "And thank them all for all their thoughts and prayers."

"Take care of yourself," Janet says. "And let me know if there is anything I can do."

—⁓—

I've promised to take Elisabeth to the cemetery, and she's looking forward to it, so I have to go. I haven't been back since the flower-kicking incident.

We stop at the discount store to pick up more flowers. I favor blue and white arrangements, but Elisabeth is partial to pinks and reds. I let her pick the flowers this time. I don't care.

I park in front of the mausoleum, and Nick's grave is only a few steps away. The grass is squishy underfoot, and I hold Elisabeth's arm so she doesn't fall. "Hi, Nicky," she says as we reach the edge of the muddy rectangle that's Nick grave.

We stand over the raw dirt in silence for a few minutes. Elisabeth likes to spend some time alone with Nick, so I say, "I'll go find the guy and remind him about the grass seed."

As I turn to walk toward the maintenance shed, I see a woman in black standing some distance away. She is standing with her head down, her face covered by the brim of her large, black hat. I've seen that hat before.

I continue on toward the maintenance shed while surreptitiously keeping my eye on that hat. I can't see the woman's face, I can't be sure if there is blond hair peeking out from below the brim. The next instant, Hat Woman is on the move. And she is moving toward Elisabeth.

She's going after Elisabeth now, I think. *Has this woman no shame?* I do an abrupt about-face. Leaping over a few headstones, I am back at Elisabeth's side in a flash. "Did you talk to the guy already?" she asks.

"Forget the guy, we have to go," I say, taking her arm, leading her firmly back to the car.

Elisabeth is confused. "Why so soon?"

"It's going to rain," I say. "I think we should get out of here."

Hat Woman has stopped a few yards from Nick's grave. Her

head is bowed as if she is praying. I help Elisabeth climb into the car and tell her to wait there for a moment.

"What are you doing here?" I shout as I walk back toward Hat Woman.

The woman looks up, startled. Her dark hair is pulled back away from her brown face. She looks scared, like I'm some sort of crazy person.

"Please excuse me," I mumble. "I'm so sorry. I thought you were someone else." I retreat back to the car, where Elisabeth is waiting.

—∿—

"So, you trashed a bouquet of flowers," Ryan says calmly, "and you yelled at a woman you don't even know. It sounds like you are feeling a lot of anger."

"You could say that," I mumble.

"Anger is a very normal part of the grieving process. You are probably also feeling abandoned, threatened, and a little scared."

"Twelve weeks ago I had a normal life. Now my husband is dead, my career is in ruins, I'm losing my son, and I think someone is stalking me. What's happening to me? Am I losing my mind?"

"Why do you believe she's stalking you?"

"Okay, so maybe it's my imagination. But what else am I imagining? Am I imagining that I am a good mother for Niko-laus? Am I imagining that I am capable of raising Matthew by myself? Am I imagining that my life was perfect before Nick died and then everything turned to crap?"

Ryan pulls some tissues out of the box on the table, hands them to me, and gives me a moment to mop the tears streaming down my face before she says, "When someone dies, it's normal to remember all the good things about that person and what it was like when they were still here. But you can take it too far. You can begin to create a fantasy past where everything was perfect, your marriage was ideal, every day was sunny."

"Like Camelot."

"Exactly." Ryan gives me a knowing look. "Jackie Kennedy was not the first or last widow to build a dream world around her late husband. But that level of perfection is hard to sustain. There will always be someone trying to push the pedestal out from under you. And you could spend the rest of your life dissatisfied that you can't replicate that dream relationship. The reality is that, like most couples, Jackie and JFK had issues."

"Very much like me and Nick."

"Very different, actually. JFK was a known philanderer. There's no reason to believe that Nick engaged in anything more than a harmless flirtation. The woman who wrote the letter to Nick may truly believe that it would have developed into something more, but that's pure speculation."

"You think I should just forget her and go on with my life."

"I think you should put her in perspective. At this point, you control the role she plays. Her fantasy life with Nick has credibility only if you believe it too. If you choose to ignore her, she'll go away. And yes, I think it's time to get on with your life. Maybe take a trip, get out of town for a while."

"She's probably already stalking her next victim," I suggest, encouraged.

"All the more reason for you to just let her go. Besides, you have two sons to concentrate on, and they need your full attention."

Reaching an
Agreement

chapter thirty-two

"**A**unt Robyn is going to call and invite us to dinner," Nikolaus says, carefully watching my reaction. "Me, you, and
Matthew."

I keep my face neutral. "That will be nice." Nikolaus's Aunt
Robyn has not spoken to me in ten years. If she's inviting me to
dinner, I can't help but wonder what she wants. Does she want to
get me on her turf so she can talk me out of the adoption? Does
she want me to see her house as proof that Nikolaus would be just
as well provided for with her?

Thanks to Nikolaus's warning, I'm not surprised when Robyn
calls the next day. "Are you free on Saturday?" she asks, acting
as if she and I invite each other to dinner all the time.

When we pull up in front of Robyn's house at the appointed
time, the Miners' car is parked in the driveway.

"Looks like Grandma Ruth is here," Nikolaus says.

Oh, joy, I think, lagging behind him up the front walk.

The last time I was at Robyn's home—ten years ago—she and her husband, Jeff, and their two children were crammed into a small apartment in a bad neighborhood. They had a large German shepherd that had the run of the place; I remember being warned to keep an eye on my dinner. But today, the address Robyn gave me on the phone turns out to be a large two-story home set back from the street in a nice residential area. As we stand at the door, I can hear a dog barking, though it sounds too youthful to be the same German shepherd.

Nikolaus told me that Robyn moved to this house about five years ago, after her youngest son was born. I had a hard time imaging the lavish digs he had described; now, as Robyn welcomes us in the marble foyer, I begin to get the picture.

Ruth Miner comes out of a doorway to greet us and then disappears. Robyn leads us into the family room, where her husband and father are seated on leather couches, watching the football game on a large-screen TV. "You can sit in here," she tells me, not so much an offer as a command. "Jeff, get Gloria a drink."

"I'm fine right now, thanks," I say.

"You have to have something to drink," Robyn says.

"No really, I'm fine. But the boys can have a soda if they want one."

"Jeff, get the boys a soda."

Jeff pushes himself out of his squashy seat and lumbers over to the mirrored bar that is built into one corner of the room. He reaches under a green marble counter and sets three cans of Coke on the counter.

"I'd stand up and say hello," LeRoy Miner says from the couch, "but I have trouble getting up from this couch."

"Please don't get up," I say sympathetically. The couches look like anyone would have trouble extracting themselves from them. Nikolaus, Matthew, and I are standing in the middle of the room, unsure what to do next.

Reaching an Agreement

"I have to finish up some things for dinner," Robyn says. "But you can make yourself at home here. Jeff, go tell the boys that Nikolaus and Matthew are here."

"Let me help you in the kitchen," I offer, as Jeff makes his way to the stairway and calls up to their boys to come downstairs. Robyn dismisses my offer with a wave of her hand.

"No, no," she says, "You just sit here and make yourself comfortable." She eyes the cans of Coke that Jeff has left on the bar with disgust. "I see you didn't get your drink yet."

"I'll get it," I say, crossing over to the bar, grateful to have something to do.

"I'll help," Nikolaus adds.

"No, I won't hear of it," Robyn insists, blocking our path to the back of the bar. "You are guests."

Nikolaus, Matthew, and I climb onto the ornate iron stools that surround the bar and watch Robyn fill three glasses with ice. Assessing the tip-over probabilities, I say, "It might be better if the kids just drink from the can." In the hands of a six-year-old, those tall glasses are an accident waiting to happen.

"No, no, no," intones Robyn, starting to pour.

Robyn's two older sons shuffle into the room. Ryan is a year older than Nikolaus, and Robbie is two years younger. They greet my kids with a "Hi" and a wave.

"Ryan, take the kids upstairs and keep them entertained until dinner," Robyn says. "I'll call you when it's ready."

Nikolaus agrees readily—he knows his cousins well and played with them often when he was younger—but Matthew is a little more hesitant. He wants to stay with me, but Robyn won't hear of it. "He'll have much more fun upstairs with the boys than down here with you," she says firmly, although from the desperate look Matthew is giving me, it is clear he doesn't agree. "You have to let your kids go sometime."

I'm shocked at her nerve in suggesting that I'm some kind of smother mother who never lets her kids out of sight. The remark also reveals her stand on the adoption, or at least that's the way I interpret it. I'm not quick-thinking enough to come back with a snappy response.

Nikolaus sees my reaction to this comment and quickly intercedes. "I need you to beat Ryan at the James Bond game," he says, grabbing Matthew's hand.

"Bring your sodas with you," Robyn commands.

Robyn's son Robbie looks troubled. "But we aren't allowed to have sodas upstairs."

"Nikolaus can be responsible for seeing that nothing gets spilled," Robyn says firmly. She gives Jeff a look, which I take to indicate that he's to go with the boys. I eye the white carpet that covers the stairs and say, "It's probably not good to be drinking sodas before dinner. Why don't you guys just leave them down here and you can have them later, when we are ready to eat?"

"That's okay," Jeff intervenes, walking behind the boys as they steady their sodas with two hands. It is obvious that further argument is futile. Robyn wins her second round. She turns her attention to me. "Go sit on the couch," she commands. "And here, take your soda."

I do as I'm told. I take the soda I didn't ask for and sink back into the soft leather. Now, with all the boys upstairs, including Jeff, I think that Robyn has created the perfect opportunity for Ruth, LeRoy, and Robyn to talk to me about the adoption. But instead Robyn retreats to the kitchen where Ruth is preparing dinner, and I'm left with LeRoy and the widescreen TV. I try to reach the coffee table to set down my glass, but I can't reach it. When I try to sit up, the couch pulls me back down. I am sitting in the middle of this huge couch, unable to move, when Jeff reappears. I try to scooch over, but it's difficult to balance the soda and scooch at the same time. Jeff sinks into the other couch, next to LeRoy, the two of them leaning away from each other as best they can.

Reaching an Agreement

Jeff and LeRoy watch the game in disinterested silence. Five minutes pass. Then ten. I don't know enough about football to attempt an intelligent comment. I consider getting up and going into the kitchen to offer to help but then decide that being stuck in the couch in silence is more pleasant than being in the kitchen with a woman who has already refused my help once and insulted my maternal abilities twice. So I sit holding my unwanted glass of Coke, which is dripping condensation into my lap.

I look around the room. It's a large room with a vaulted ceiling. The furniture is obviously new and looks like it was selected by a decorator. There are all the professional touches you would expect to find in a nice hotel lobby—expensive but somehow cold. Would Nikolaus be happy living here?

I wonder how Jeff and Robyn can afford this house. Jeff works for his dad, who is an accountant. Robyn works a few days a week as a secretary in her father's office. Seeing the way they live, it's obvious that their parents have given them much more than just jobs. I seem to recall that Jeff has a brother and maybe a sister, too, so it's unlikely that Jeff's parents paid for this house. It's more likely that since Rachael's death, Robyn has become the "alpha daughter," the recipient of everything the Miners wish they could have given to Rachael, if only she had lived. I wonder how Rob Miner feels about his parents' largesse toward his sister. Maybe that's why he's not here tonight. Rob's law practice earns him a decent but by no means spectacular living. He lives in a modest house and we've talked about the financial challenges of putting three kids through college. Suddenly the underlying level of tension I've always felt existed between he and Robyn makes perfect sense.

I wonder what Nick would think about all this. Nick, who worked hard to earn everything he ever had. Would Nick want his son to live in a place, however nice, where nothing had been earned?

Hanging over the fireplace is one of those large family portraits that looks like it was shot through a lens covered in Vaseline. Robyn is standing over Jeff, who is sitting in a wing chair. The kids are arranged in what looks like uncomfortable positions at his feet. There is a dog, but it's not a German shepherd. If Nikolaus came to live here, would they take a new picture to include him?

I notice that there are half a dozen framed pictures on the mantel. One is of Rachael, dressed in a hospital gown and looking very pale, leaning over an incubator that holds a newly born Nikolaus. Rachael is touching one of his tiny hands, careful not to disturb the network of tubes and wires attached to every other part of his tiny body. Another photo is of Rachael and Robyn as young girls, sitting on a couch and smiling into the camera. There is a formal portrait of Rachael in her wedding gown and a picture of Rachael climbing out of a pool. Except for the formal family portrait, there are no pictures of Robyn's children and no pictures of her husband. Every picture on the mantel is of Rachael. I wonder if she puts those pictures out only when Nikolaus is coming or if she has them out all the time.

Robyn comes in and announces it is time to eat. "I'll put this on the table for you," she says, grabbing my glass. Mercifully, this allows me the use of two hands to extract myself from the couch.

Dinner is an uneventful progression of roast beef, mashed potatoes, and glazed carrots served on silver platters and china dishes. The conversation consists of the adults asking the children a series of questions. We discover what grades the kids are in, what their favorite and least favorite subjects are, and what they are planning for the future. Jeff keeps my wine glass full, which is not hard to do because I take only tiny sips. I am beginning to wonder if I've been worrying all night for nothing. Maybe Robyn invited me because she wanted to get to know me better, after all these years. She had an opportunity to discuss the adoption before dinner, but she didn't. On the other hand, if this dinner was an excuse to deliver bad news, she would definitely wait until after dinner to do it. So I continue to pretend to drink my wine and focus on keeping my guard up.

In the break between dinner and dessert, the boys are allowed to disappear back upstairs. The men return to the TV, and I insist on helping to clear the dishes. I gingerly stack the delicate china on the polished granite counter next to the sink while Ruth busily makes coffee. Robyn is rearranging the leftovers in the side-by-side stainless steel refrigerator. There is no conversation. I offer to load the dishes into the dishwasher, but Robyn shoos me away. "Those dishes need to be done by hand," she says. "Jeff and Ryan will do them later."

Robyn brings mugs of coffee out to the men in the family room and then sets the kitchen table with three cups and saucers, teaspoons, and napkins. I guess that a little klatch is planned for Ruth, Robyn, and me. I'm sure that this is when the real agenda for the evening will be revealed. This is where the rubber meets the road. My stomach reflexively clenches and for a moment I think I might throw up. *I'm not up to this,* I think. I can't stand up for myself against Ruth and Robyn. I can't stand up for Nikolaus. I just want to go home.

"I'm so glad that you could come tonight," Robyn says, settling herself at the table. "We've been meaning to have you and the boys over for a long time."

Like ten years? I think, but I say, "Thanks so much for having us. It's been lovely."

Ruth says, "The time after a death is always so difficult. We know exactly what you are going through." Robyn nods vigorously.

I don't ask how they could possibly know what I am going through when their husbands sit, very much alive, watching the game in the next room. But I sip my coffee and say nothing.

Robyn continues, "I have no doubt that you'll come through this just fine. I've always said that you were an amazing woman." Now Ruth is nodding.

Maybe it's just a reaction to the tension I'm feeling, but this statement is so patently ridiculous that I almost laugh. Then I start to get pissed off. Do they really expect me to believe that they've been thinking of me all these years as "amazing"? I decide it's time to stop being nice. "Frankly, I'm surprised to hear you say that. I always thought that you didn't like me much."

Robyn's eyes widen in an expression of surprise that does not look genuine at all. "Oh, no," she says. "I've always admired you. I'm just sorry that we couldn't be better friends because of the difficulties with Nick."

"Difficulties?"

"I made a promise to Rachael that I would always watch out for Nikolaus," Robyn says. "Nick did many things that went against Rachael's wishes. But I don't blame you for that."

I'm confused. "You mean while Rachael was alive?"

"Nick couldn't take care of Rachael," Ruth says. "He was busy with his own concerns. He was really a very selfish person."

Nick was not a perfect person, but selfish he was not. How dare she criticize Nick? Ruth can see that I am offended and hastily adds, "Of course, Nick had many good qualities. He was a good father for the most part. But I know that Rachael would have wanted us to be more involved in Nikolaus's life. Nick was against that for some reason."

Controlling my anger, I choose my words carefully. "I'm sure that Nick did what he felt was best for Nikolaus."

Robyn, oblivious to my clenched jaw, continues in a dreamy voice, "I remember the day after Rachael died. I was sitting at home, drinking coffee, just like we are now. And Rachael came and sat down with me and told me how much better she felt, that all the pain was gone, and that she could rest now as long as she knew that I would take care of Nikolaus. Nikolaus was her only concern."

She has my full attention now. I forget to be angry. "Rachael came to see you?" I ask. "She came after she died?"

"Oh, yes," Robyn says. "She was so concerned about Nikolaus, she couldn't rest."

"She was a devoted mother," Ruth agrees, wiping her eyes, "and a wonderful person."

"A saint," Robyn says, patting Ruth's hand.

"So did she only come that once?" I ask. "Did she ever come again?"

"Oh, she speaks to me often," Robyn says. "Even now, I often feel her presence. And, of course, now Nick is with her, too. I like to think that they are together at last."

The picture of Nick and Rachael happily together in heaven is not one I want to spend a whole lot of time thinking about, especially when I'm down here trying to deal with Ruth and Robyn.

"I like to think that Rachael rests in peace," Ruth says. "But she has definite feelings on how she would like Nikolaus to be raised."

Suddenly, I think I know where this is going. I've heard this argument from Ruth before in various versions. Rachael would want Nikolaus to spend Christmas with the Miners. Rachael would want Nikolaus to go to the Catholic school that is conveniently located near Robyn's house and twenty miles from ours. Rachael would want Nikolaus to spend his birthday weekend at the Miners' cabin, which Nick and I were not invited to. Nick could stand up to them. Nick had the right to do what was truly best for Nikolaus, regardless of "what Rachael would want." Now, I'm sure "what Rachael would want" is for Nikolaus to live with Ruth—or with Robyn. Without Nick, I'm not sure I can fight them. I feel cold, clammy.

Ruth says, "I've talked with Nikolaus about his future. As you know, I am ready to rent an apartment near his school if he wants to finish school with his class. Or, he could come live here with Robyn and Jeff and be part of their family. There is an excellent Catholic school here. Obviously, he would be very welcome and well cared for."

Robyn is nodding vigorously. "We would raise him as one of our own."

I can't speak, I can't react. I can just sit and wait for them to finish. Ruth continues, "We all know that you have been a good . . ." She chokes on the word "mother." ". . . influence on Nikolaus. Now, he seems to feel strongly that he wants to stay with you through this difficult time. I think he feels an obligation to you, and to Matthew."

Obligation. This is the same word Kathy used. When did I become such an obligation to everyone?

"He's grown into such a responsible young man," Robyn tells Ruth, congratulating her as if it were all her doing.

Ruth takes a deep breath and stiffens her neck as if she is about to say something difficult, something painful. "In light of Nikolaus's feelings, LeRoy and I have decided that it is in Nikolaus's best interest that we agree to your adopting him," she says. "I thought it would be best to tell you in person."

I'm sure that I did not hear her correctly. "I don't understand," I say. "Can you please repeat that?"

"We invited you here tonight to tell you that we will sign the adoption papers," Robyn says. "It's what Nikolaus seems to want."

To say I am surprised by her words is a gross understatement. I have been steeling myself all night, waiting for her to say exactly the opposite. "I don't know what to say. Thank you, Ruth. Thank you so much."

"Tell your lawyer to send the papers to Rob. He'll look the agreement over and then we'll sign it." Ruth looks as though she has aged ten years in the last half hour. In all the time I've known her, I've had a lot of strong feeling toward her, but now, for the first time, I mostly feel sorry for her. I know that agreeing to sign the adoption papers is one of the most difficult things she will ever do, a Solomon's choice in which she might lose her grandson either way. "I know how hard this decision is for you," I say to her.

"We'll still be involved in Nikolaus's life," Robyn interjects quickly. "We are still his family, and nothing will ever change that."

"I'll still be watching you," Ruth warns. "Now, let's get those boys some pie."

—⚏—

I'm relieved that Ruth Miner has agreed to sign the adoption papers, but I know I'm not home free. Nick's will names Rob Miner as Nikolaus's legal guardian. I had put all my energy into worrying about Ruth Miner because she was the bigger obstacle. But for the adoption to sail through uncontested, I still need Rob Miner on my side.

I have always felt that Rob could be an ally to me in dealing with the Miners, although I haven't had the opportunity to test this theory until now. Nick and Rob remained friends of a sort, even after the split with the Miners. And in the days after Nick died, Rob stopped by the house once or twice, just to see if there was anything he could do. I was too shaken at the time to talk to him about the adoption, but now it seems that he will be the one looking over the documents and ensuring that things go smoothly between me and his parents.

Rob immediately accepts my offer to come for coffee when I call him the next morning after the dinner.

Two mornings later, we settle in the kitchen—he with coffee, I with my chamomile tea—and I get right to the point. "When

Nick and I were first married, we went to a lawyer and had wills prepared," I say. "After Matthew was born, we updated those wills, but unfortunately, we never signed them."

I feel like I'm talking gibberish, and Rob looks confused. I plunge ahead. "The bottom line is that Nick's first will, the one that's still legally valid, named you as Nikolaus's guardian."

Rob's reaction is not what I expected. "Nick named *me*?" he asks, his eyes filling with tears. "Wow, what an honor."

"You didn't know that? Nick didn't tell you?"

"No, he never said anything. When Rachael was alive, Nick and I were pretty tight. Nick needed a friend in the family, so to speak, because my mom and sister can be pretty rough, as you know. But I never thought that he would name me as guardian."

He's acting like he just won the lottery. I was thinking that this would be an easy conversation, but now I am not so sure. Does this mean he wants Nikolaus?

"I think Nick knew that you would do what was best for Nikolaus," I say. When Rob and his wife were together and their kids were younger, they were a good choice to raise Nikolaus. But now Rob and his wife aren't together, and Nikolaus has a brother. Nick's updated—but unsigned—will names me as Nikolaus's guardian if I were to survive Nick, and his cousin Tom as legal guardian for both boys if Nick and I were both to die. But I don't go into that with Rob now. It's all a moot point anyway. As the lawyer said, you can't will away your children.

Rob looks at me somberly. "I know that my mother tried to get Nikolaus to choose between you and her. I told her she was wrong to do that."

Now it's my turn to get teary. "Thank you," I whisper. "Thank you so much." I take a deep breath and continue. "You know that I had dinner with your mother and Robyn," I tell him. "And they said you would look over the papers for them before they signed."

Reaching an Agreement

Rob sits back down, looking thoughtful. He wraps his hands around his coffee mug and studies it for a long moment before he speaks, ignoring the issue I just addressed. "I didn't know that Nick gave me the responsibility of being Nikolaus's guardian. I have great respect for Nick, and I respect his choice." Rob takes a sip of coffee, then continues, "Nick named me as guardian because he trusted me to do what is best for Nikolaus. Nick was a good man and a good friend. I won't let him down." I start to feel my stomach lunge and I realize that Rob and I are not on the same page regarding this visit.

"So you're saying that you want to adopt Nikolaus?" I ask. It's a gut reaction. It's my worst fear.

Rob looks at me in surprise. "Why would I want to do that?" he asks, genuinely bewildered. "I told you, I want to do what's best for him. You're Nikolaus's mom. What's best for him is for him to stay here with you and Matthew. I thought I was here to look over the papers and discuss how dinner at my sister's house went. I'm on your side." I settle back down with my chamomile tea and decide that it's finally time to let go of the paranoia that's been haunting me for so many months.

A Needed Vacation

chapter thirty-three

I can't breathe.

Air goes in and out of my lungs, but I still feel like I'm suffocating, like there's an elephant sitting on my chest. It's been happening on and off for weeks, maybe longer. At first I thought it was an allergy or asthma, so I didn't worry about it too much. Then for a few days I thought I had lung cancer, but since I wasn't coughing, I figured I was safe. This morning, my chest feels tight, and I think I'm having a heart attack.

I sit in the doctor's waiting room reading an outdated *People*. A smartly dressed woman walks up to the receptionist and loudly announces, "I am here for my eleven o'clock appointment," employing a tone that says they better not keep her waiting. I remember when I used to be that demanding, that self-important. It seems like a hundred years ago. Now I sit and wait patiently, trying to catch my breath.

"It'll be just a few minutes," the receptionist tells her. "We have a patient who is having chest pains and needs to be seen right away." The receptionist motions to me, and the woman with the eleven o'clock appointment eyes me suspiciously. I drop *People* on the table and follow the receptionist through the white door.

They take my temperature, measure my blood pressure, extract two vials of blood from my arm, and ask me to blow repeatedly into a tube. While I'm waiting for the doctor's entrance, I notice that my chest is not as constricted as before. I'm starting to feel better. I'm starting to feel stupid about coming here.

The doctor comes in with a clipboard and a folder that I recognize as my medical records. I've averaged one visit here a month for the past four months: I poked my eye and came in for pain medication, then I came because I was having trouble with double vision, which turned out to be a symptom of exhaustion. And I was here twice last month, convinced that I had breast cancer.

"Your blood chemistry is normal," the doctor says, "and you seem to have good lung function."

"I'm actually feeling a little bit better now," I say. "But this morning I thought I was having a heart attack."

He listens to my heart, my breathing. He thumps my chest and my back. He even hooks me up to an EKG machine and carefully watches the jumping needles while assuring me that it is rare for pre-menopausal women to have heart problems.

"You've been under a lot of stress," he says. "I know you are against taking antidepressants. But maybe you should consider taking a break. A small vacation might do you a lot of good right now."

At least it will keep me out of his office.

—⚍—

The kids are out of school for the summer, and we have no plans. Maybe we do need a change of scenery.

"How about we go on vacation?" I suggest to the kids.

"I don't want to go," Matthew says immediately.

Nikolaus slips easily into the role of peacemaker. "You don't even know where we are going yet," he says. "We could go somewhere really fun."

Matthew crosses his arms. "I don't want to have fun."

Nikolaus sighs.

My mother calls me every Sunday. "You and the boys should get away," she encourages. "Why don't you come home and see your family?" In a moment of weakness, I agree. Even though Elisabeth lives on her own, I don't feel comfortable leaving for two or three weeks without her. She doesn't love the idea, either. "If you guys die on the plane, I don't want to be left alone," she tells me. So I invite her to come along.

When we arrive in New York, the temperature is 95 degrees with 98 percent humidity. Waiting for the rental car at Kennedy, I feel like I'm in a steam bath. The oppressive heat is not helping my breathing problems at all, but I don't want to alarm the kids, so I pretend that I'm feeling just fine.

My uncles live ten minutes from the airport. When the wind is right, the noise from the planes landing interrupts conversations and forces you to turn up the volume on the TV. Today, though, their house is quiet except for the hum of the window air conditioner.

My Uncle Babe spent forty years in the restaurant business, and today he's prepared a spread that proves it: cold poached salmon, fresh corn, tomato-and-mozzarella salad, and chocolate cake. "You don't want a real drink," Vincent says, pouring me a glass of iced tea. "You still have to drive."

I ask Elisabeth if she wants to go lie down, but she says she prefers to sit at the table with us. The fact that the boys ate lunch and snacked on the plane does not stop them from eating again. "Everybody looks healthy," Babe says with satisfaction, watching them. "God bless."

The uncles ask Elisabeth what she hears from her sister in Germany. They ask about the Miners' health. Nikolaus, of course, doesn't mention that his grandmother had called him just before we left to ask if I was forcing him to move to New York. And I am not admitting to anyone, myself included, that this trip might be a good chance for me to see if moving back home—nearer to family and cheaper housing—might not be such a bad alternative.

"Call your mother," Vincent says to me. "She'll be worried."

"You better get on the road soon," my mother warns when I call her. "I don't want you to drive after dark."

The uncles won't be talked out of packing sandwiches and sodas for the trip even though the drive to Pennsylvania will take no more than three hours and we have just eaten. They also provide a map and detailed directions, although it is a trip I've taken hundreds of times and could probably do blindfolded.

Once in the car, I decide on a whim to cut through the city instead of taking the more direct route through Brooklyn and over the Verrazano Bridge. *We're explorers, here to see the sights,* I think as we head across the Long Island Expressway toward the Midtown Tunnel. *We are starting a grand adventure.*

In the city, Saturday-night traffic is light, and I make a quick swing up Sixth Avenue past Rockefeller Center to Central Park. The hansom cabs line up at the park entrance, but Matthew is less interested in the horses than I expect. We head back downtown on Fifth past St. Patrick's Cathedral and the great lions of the Public Library.

Matthew perks up as we pass the Empire State Building. "Can we go up to the top?" he begs. "Please?" But parking is difficult, and I'm afraid that Elisabeth can't make the trip to the top.

"Another time," I promise.

South of Houston, the streets of the financial district are largely deserted, and we swing past the World Trade Center and head toward the building on Maiden Lane where my father worked for many years and the restaurant on Pearl that my grandfather owned, which was sold out of the family years ago. These last sights are included in the tour for my benefit; I don't expect they will make much of an impression on the boys or Elisabeth. But they are touchstones for me, vague memories of a distant past, the starting points from which I can measure how far I've come.

Matthew is fascinated by lower Manhattan. "Do they make money there?" he asks as we pass the Stock Exchange. "Do they let people live here?" He remains glued to the window as we head back up toward the Holland Tunnel.

It is almost nine o'clock when we arrive at my mother's house. We find her in tears. "Where have you been?" she sobs. "I've been frantic."

I decide it's better not to mention the detour through the city—which, in any case, added no more than an hour to the trip.

"I've called the highway patrol several times," my mother goes on. "I had visions of you all lying dead on the side of the road."

It's going to be a long three weeks.

After a week of visiting with my mother and sisters, the boys and I pack up and head to Stone Harbor, on the Jersey shore. We leave Elisabeth with my mother—she doesn't like sun, sand, or swimming, and I need a break from being fussed over by older ladies.

"Can we stop at the Empire State Building on the way?" Matthew asks, but I explain that we're going the opposite direction.

I head out with high hopes. I long to escape the oppressive humidity and breathe in cool ocean breezes. As a child, I spent a week each summer at the shore, and I was anxious to share this experience with my children: Swimming in the buoyant saltwater. Riding the gentle waves into shore. Feeling the sandy grit between my toes, in the crotch of my bathing suit. Hearing the cut-rate calliope music and the clack of the roller coaster, bathing in the boardwalk's neon lights.

I had originally thought of going to Cape May, but I knew the kids wouldn't enjoy the quaint bed-and-breakfasts that predominate there. I settled instead on the town of Stone Harbor because I remembered it as being more family-oriented.

"I don't know what kind of hotel you'll find down there," my sister had warned. "Most people rent houses." Indeed, the hotel I booked is far less comfortable than I had hoped. The room is so small that the two double beds butt against one another, but the bathroom is clean and there is a small slice of ocean view from the three-foot-wide balcony. Plus, I don't have to cook meals, and the maid comes daily to make the beds and provide fresh towels, so it feels like a real vacation.

We pin the temporary beach badges the hotel provides on our swimsuits and head down to the shore, which is blazing hot and suspiciously empty. "Isn't this great?" I chirp. "We have the whole beach to ourselves."

"My feet are burning up," Matthew complains, "and there is a lot of gross stuff down by the water."

Great clear blobs dot the sand at the water's edge and jiggle in the ebbing tide. Nikolaus stoops to investigate. "Jellyfish," he declares. "Millions of them."

"Cool!" Matthew pokes tentatively at one with his finger. "Can we eat them?"

"Don't touch it!" I shout, pulling his hand back. "It will sting you," I explain, more calmly.

We retreat to the hotel pool, which is where we find the crowd. The pool is very small and full of chubby, sunburned children. All the lounge chairs are already occupied by women in gold lamé or rhinestone-studded swimsuits and red manicured nails. They are all coiffed and wearing eye makeup. "This is half the size of our pool at home," Matthew complains, "and it has twice as many people."

"But there's waitress service," I say, trying to make the best of a bad situation. I order frosty drinks for the kids and sit on the side of the pool, dangling my feet in the filmy, lukewarm water, sipping my mai tai. The kids go in the pool just long enough to get wet, then decide to go back up to the room and watch TV. I order another drink and spread my towel on the concrete behind a row of lounging women, far enough from the splashing crowd to stay dry but close enough to hear the distant sound of the waves and eavesdrop on the women's conversations. I am breathing easier.

"Harry's played golf for three days in a row," one lady whines to another. "Meanwhile, I'm stuck with the kids."

A bleached blond is saying, "I think I'll go to the outlet mall tomorrow, even if I have to lock the kids in the room. I hear they have Gucci."

Her friend says, "I'm going with you, and I'm going to buy myself something really nice. That schmuck I married is going to pay. He was supposed to take the kids to get ice cream three hours ago."

My chances of joining in on a conversation with these women are slim to none. What would we have in common? They sound like they want to kill their husbands. I just buried mine. We have different goals. I came here hoping to spend time with my kids, and they came here hoping to escape them. I leave my drink unfinished and head up to the room to see what my boys are doing.

I had planned to stay at the beach for four days, but by day three, we've all had enough and are ready to leave. We've played miniature golf on a small course on the roof of a gift shop, bought T-shirts, eaten cotton candy, and spent at least twice the money on carnival games than the few prizes we've won would have cost at full retail. We spent an entire day on the boardwalk, riding the log flume, the twister, the bumper cars, and the haunted house. We rode four different roller coasters, twice each.

As we're leaving the boardwalk, Matthew begs for one last ride. There is a small steel roller coaster, a kiddy ride, near the exit. Nikolaus says he's had enough, so I climb into the small car with Matthew. On the first turn, the car abruptly turns sideways, and I am jostled against the side. I feel something snap. A sharp pain shoots through my side and is exacerbated by every twist and turn we take. My screams of pain blend seamlessly into the joyful screams from other riders.

Back at the hotel, I look for a bruise, but there is none. Based on the level of pain, I figure I must have cracked a rib. Breathing is now not only difficult, it's painful. I wish that Nick were here to take care of me. He'd go to the drugstore for me and get me some Tylenol. He'd be the one walking up and down the aisles right now looking for some kind of bandage or brace that would ease the pain so that I could drive home. I wish that Nick were here to drive us back to my mother's, but he's not. Nikolaus loads the luggage in the car. I stay in the slow lane of the turnpike the entire way back, trying to keep my torso still, hoping that I won't have to make any sudden painful turns.

We get back to my mother's house in the late afternoon. She's upset because I didn't call her every day while we were at the shore.

"We were only gone for three days," I protest.

"You should have called to let us know that you were still alive," my mother says stiffly. "Elisabeth and I were out of our minds with worry." The two of them sit at the dining room table drinking coffee and eating apple cake. Apparently, all the worry hasn't affected their appetite.

"I live three thousand miles away and don't call you every day. I'm sorry, but it never occurred to me to call you daily from fifty miles away."

My mother takes another bite of cake and then continues as if I hadn't spoken, "And you never even called to tell us when you were coming back. Now the kids are probably starving, and I have no dinner ready."

"Don't worry. We ate some burgers on the way."

She ignores me, focusing her attention on Elisabeth. "Luckily we have a lasagna in the refrigerator. I know the kids love lasagna."

"Thanks, Mom. That will be just perfect." What else can I say?

A Distasteful Dinner

chapter thirty-four

We are home less than a week when Nikolaus says, "Maybe we should invite Aunt Robyn and Uncle Jeff over for dinner."

I am not enthused about the idea, but he looks so hopeful that I have to agree. "I'll call them and ask when they can come."

Robyn puts me off for weeks. We set a date, but then Jeff has to go out of town, so they cancel. We change the date, but then Robyn has to work that day. Then the family comes down with the flu. I keep trying because it seems to mean a lot to Nikolaus that they come. Finally, Robyn agrees to come have dinner with us, but only if she can bring pizza. I'm too exasperated to argue with her.

They show up with three pizzas. Nikolaus is anxious to show Ryan and Robbie around the house. Although Nikolaus has invited the boys over many times for birthday parties or just to hang out with him, this is the first time they've actually been to the house.

Nikolaus wants so much for everyone to get along, for all of us to have a nice time together. I open a bottle of wine for the adults and offer soft drinks to the kids.

"So, are you going to be able to stay in this house?" Robyn asks while I'm passing out the plates. Although it's an obvious question, no one has asked me this so bluntly in the months since Nick's death. I try not to let the fact that I'm offended show in my response. "At least until Nikolaus graduates from high school," I say. "After that, we'll see."

Nikolaus jumps in. "We did a lot of work on this house ourselves," he says proudly. "Papa and I did a lot of stuff together."

"Well, it's probably too much work for Gloria to handle," Robyn says to Nikolaus, "and too much money." This may be true, but I don't appreciate her saying it out loud, or to Nikolaus, for that matter.

"Don't worry," I assure him, "we'll manage."

"It's not the kind of house your mother would like," Robyn continues, "but I guess it's home now."

Jeff, sensing trouble, excuses himself from the table without explanation. Nikolaus looks uncomfortable, waiting for me to explode. But I'm not giving Robyn the satisfaction of making me mad.

"It is our home," I say, "and we have no plans to leave it."

We eat for a while in silence. Jeff comes back to the table, smelling of soap. He avoids looking at me.

Finished with their pizza, the boys excuse themselves, and Nikolaus takes them upstairs to listen to music and play video games. I'm left alone with Robyn and Jeff. When Robyn suggests watching a movie, I gratefully agree. At least it will head off any further uncomfortable conversation.

They leave shortly after the movie ends. The kids are reluctant to leave; they are having a good time together. Nikolaus hugs Ryan and Robbie at the door. "Come back, man," he says. "Soon."

"Thanks for having them over," Nikolaus says to me after they leave. "I had a great time. Did you?"

"Well, it was interesting," I say. Unlike Nikolaus, I hope that they *don't* come back soon.

Better Than Therapy

chapter thirty-five

One of my earliest memories is of my parents arguing over money. My father staunchly refused to go into debt, aside from taking out the mortgage, which he viewed as his personal ball and chain. Living within our means meant few luxuries—our furniture was largely secondhand, vacations were a few days in a rooming house down at the shore, and our family car was a ten-year-old Chevy, a hand-me-down from the uncles. If we mentioned that our friends watched color televisions, rented shore houses for an entire month, or rode in newer cars, my father's inevitable response would be, "We don't have *that kind* of money." I was nearly a teenager before I realized that there weren't actually different kinds of money. Until then, I thought that our family only got the kind of money used to buy sensible shoes, sturdy wool coats, and meatloaf, not the kind that could buy patent leather, fake fur, or T-bone steaks.

Now I am wondering what kind of money I have. I know now that I don't want to move to the East Coast, but can I afford to stay in California? I don't have enough to get rid of the mortgage, but should I pay it down? I have enough to send to Nikolaus to college, but will there be enough left in ten more years, when it's Matthew's turn? Ever since Nick died, my career has been in neutral, even reverse. How long can I continue to coast before I get down to serious work again? Should I start looking for a full-time job?

"I took my mother to see a financial advisor after my father died," Janine tells me. "He helped her organize her finances and figure out a budget for living expenses. But that was in Arizona."

The next time I meet with Jerry to discuss the adoption, I check out the names on the other doors in his office. One is listed as an investment advisor, but I don't need advice on investing, I need advice on spending. When I ask about the person with the title "Financial Consultant" under her name, the receptionist confides, "She only works three days a week, and all her clients have a least a million dollars."

Schwab has a division that works with financial advisors and I ask Melanie for information about their services. She sets up a meeting with a Schwab person in the Montgomery Street branch. A few phone calls later, I have an appointment with a financial advisor who has agreed to do a financial plan for me for what seems like a reasonable price. And her office is located in Orinda, the town right next to where I live.

The woman's office is in a small, two-story building with a fountain in the courtyard. She asks me to bring current bank statements, mortgage receipts, and utility bills to our first meeting. We discuss what she calls "life scenarios." One is that I go back to work full-time next year and continue living in our current house. Another is that I sell the house after Nikolaus graduates high school and move to a cheaper house. The scenario I'm rooting for is the one where I stay in our house and work part-time, which is what I'm doing now.

In three weeks, I'm back in her office to hear the results. Computer-printed spreadsheets that detail estimated income and expenses, including fictitious but inevitable home repairs, are spread across the oak table in her office. She explains that each scenario we discussed has been carried through a fifty-year period, after which I will be over ninety years old, and includes adjustments for inflation, escalating medical expenses, and growth on investments I don't yet own. The detail is exhausting. "What's the bottom line?" I ask.

"If you stay in your current house, working part-time as you are now, I estimate that you will run out of money in twenty or thirty years. You'll be sixty-five and living off Social Security, which I wouldn't recommend." She pulls out another spreadsheet. "If you stay in your current house and work full-time, you'll be seventy by the time you have to live off Social Security."

"I only get five additional years from working full-time?" I ask.

"If you are working full-time, I assumed increased expenses for transportation, daycare, and clothes. If you can cap those expenses, you may eke out a few additional years."

"Where's the scenario where I live happily ever after?" I ask.

She pulls out the last spreadsheet. "This is the one that I would recommend," she says. "You keep your current house for another two years until Nikolaus finishes high school. Then you sell it and move to something less expensive. Maybe it's not as big as your current house, or maybe it's in a lower-cost area. With your mortgage payment reduced, you may only have to work full-time for another ten years, or work part-time and retire at sixty-five. Either way, you can plan on celebrating your ninetieth birthday with cash to spare."

As she is speaking, I feel like a weight is being lifted slowly off my shoulders, and when she finishes, I feel happy and peaceful. This is better than any therapy session I've ever had. This is like a trip to the ultimate psychic. For the first time since Nick died, I begin to feel hopeful about the future.

No Place Like Home

chapter thirty-six

My lawyer, Jerry, had told me to be prepared for a visit from the Child Welfare Department, so when the man calls on a Wednesday morning and asks if he can come over that afternoon, I'm not surprised.

I spend the rest of the morning making sure the house is clean and tidy. I make the beds, straighten the towels in the bathroom, and sweep the kitchen floor. I kick the toys that litter the floor in Matthew's room under his bed and arrange the bedspread to cover them. Nikolaus keeps his room in military order, so there's nothing for me to do in there. And though I doubt that the Child Welfare officer will inspect my office, I arrange the drift of papers on my desk into neat piles to give the impression of organization and efficiency.

Promptly at 2:00 PM, a small, bespectacled man presents himself at the front door. He is wearing an ill-fitting polyester jacket over a rumpled polo shirt and khakis. I have put on dark wool slacks and a cashmere sweater, trying to look casual yet conservative.

I show him into the living room, but he asks if there is a table we can use. There is paperwork to be done, he explains. We sit in the dining room. He accepts my offer of the coffee that I have just made, the smell of it wafting through the house. I bring out a plate of store-bought cookies; baking my own would have been a bit over the top.

"Tell me about yourself," he says, and I do. I tell him I'm self-employed but have steady work, and I name some well-known companies that have been clients. He has a pad of paper, and he writes down the names of the companies. "How much do you earn in an average year?" he asks, and he writes that down, too. He asks if I am expecting any financial benefit from adopting Nikolaus, access to trust funds or future inheritances, that sort of thing. "He has a college fund," I say, "and I get a monthly check for him from Social Security."

"I bet Social Security is not covering the mortgage on this place," he says, smiling.

"Actually, I'll probably have to sell this house," I say, and then hasten to add, "but not until after Nikolaus graduates from high school." I am happy to see him making a note of this.

"Were you born in California?" he asks.

"No. New Jersey," I say.

"Where?"

"A small town up north."

"What's the name of it?"

"Somerville."

Can you spell that?" I do. He writes it down and then asks, "How long did you live there?"

"Until I was about two years old."

He writes that down. "Then where did you go?"

I tell him. I spell the names of every place I've ever lived, every school I've ever gone to, every company I've ever worked for. He writes it all down.

"Have you ever been convicted of a felony?" he asks. "Have you ever been arrested for child molestation, child endangerment, or child neglect? Are you currently enrolled in an educational, training, or rehabilitation program of any kind? Are you currently using any illegal substances on a regular or occasional basis?"

I shake my head to each question he poses.

"How many alcoholic drinks have you had today?"

"None. I don't really drink."

He writes it all down. He asks more questions. Then he asks me to sign a statement saying that all the information I have given him is true and that I understand that the state of California will check out everything I've said. He asks me if I want to change anything I've told him before I sign.

"I was hoping to meet briefly with Nikolaus today," he says when we're finished with the paperwork, looking at his watch. "What time does he get home from school?"

"Should be any minute," I tell him. It is already after three. "What are the next steps in this process? I mean, after you check out everything I've said . . ."

"Once the investigation is complete, then I'll publish a final report," he says. "You'll get a copy, and a copy will go to the judge."

"How long will the investigation take?" I ask.

"Your lawyer has petitioned the court to expedite the process. If the juvenile adoption process isn't completed by the time Nikolaus is eighteen, then you'll have to apply to adopt him as an adult. That means you'll have to start all over from the beginning."

"But he's only sixteen. That gives us two years. That's plenty of time, isn't it?"

He shakes his head. "An adoption like this, where the kid is in a nice home with a stable parent, can drag on for years, mostly because there is no urgency to complete it. Our priorities are cases where the kids are living in filth or in dangerous situations. That's where I spend most of my time. I don't spend much time in houses like this, checking out what college the parent went to." He sighs and finishes the last sip of his coffee. "Most times, it's good that it's a slow process. It gives the birth parents time to get their act together, if they are going to. And it gives the adoptive parents time to understand what they are getting into. Once the adoption is final, it's forever. There is no going back."

"I know exactly what I'm getting into," I tell him. "I've been Nikolaus's mother for ten years."

The front door opens, and I can hear Nikolaus's voice trading banter with his friend Sean. When they enter the kitchen, they see us sitting in the dining room. "What's up?" Nikolaus asks.

I introduce Nikolaus, explaining the man is from Child Welfare. "Actually, I work for the juvenile court," he corrects me. "I'm a probation officer." He stands and shakes hands with Nikolaus and with Sean. "I'd like to take a few minutes to talk to you if I could," he says to Nikolaus.

"I gotta go anyway," Sean says, backing out the door.

The probation officer suggests they talk up in Nikolaus's room. "Call if you need me," I say, more to Nikolaus than to the officer. I wouldn't normally allow a stranger to be in my son's room alone, but in this case, I don't feel I can object.

The officer comes down the stairs a half hour later. "He's a very nice kid," he says, handing me his card. "I'll do what I can to speed things up for both of you." I see him to the door.

"He asked to see my clothes, my books, my video games, my homework," Nikolaus tells me when the officer has gone. "He asked what I thought of you being my mother, and he asked about Matthew and about Papa. He asked if there was anyplace else I'd rather live than here, and I told him no, I wanted to stay here."

"And what did he say to that?" I asked.

"He said that he wouldn't mind living in a place like this, either."

Unexpected Help

chapter thirty-seven

Doug never called me again after that last meeting. I think he's probably hired someone else to finish the project. I called Stephen, the art director who brought me in, to find out what was going on. He said Doug hasn't called him either, but he may have been trying to spare my feelings.

I met with Melanie a few days after that last meeting with Doug.

"I have something I want you to work on," Melanie said. "I need an analysis of the results for last year's direct mail programs. I think you are the perfect person to do it."

"I want you to spend some time digging into the data," Melanie said. "There's no real deadline; anything you find out will be helpful. Just work on it whenever you can."

The company Melanie works for is a high-pressure, high-profile financial firm, so I knew something was up. "There are no projects without deadlines here," I said. "Do you think I can't handle a real project?"

"I think you may not realize how hard Nick's death has hit you," Melanie said, "or how long the effects of it are going to last. Three years ago, my sister died in a car accident. I was a mess for months—I couldn't sleep, I couldn't eat, I had trouble concentrating. I'm still not over it completely. I can only imagine what you are going through."

"Really, I'm fine," I said. "I'm ready to get back to work."

"Then do this project for me. Look, I really need this analysis done and no one else has the time to do it. There is an office here you can work in. Come in when you can, work when you're able, and keep me up to date on any results as you find them."

The project turns out to be somewhat tedious, as it requires sorting through mail samples, response data, and account records. It does not require quick decisions, persuasive arguments, or multilevel strategies—things I used to be really good at, but now seem as impossible to me as suddenly speaking a foreign language or playing professional sports. The project does, however, give me a reason to get dressed and out of the house three or four days a week, and it keeps my mind occupied. I am grateful to Melanie.

In the first few days, I don't get much done—not because I'm having trouble concentrating but because several times a day, I look up from my work to find someone standing in my office doorway. Some are people I've worked with, others are people I know only by sight. They come into my cubicle to offer condolences or to volunteer help. Sometimes they sit down in the extra chair and we talk. A surprising number of them tell me stories about someone close to them who has died. These are not people I know well—most, I hardly know at all. But they know my story, and they feel compelled to share theirs with me. They feel that it will help me. They feel they can trust me. They feel I'll understand.

Their stories are sometimes terrible—a parent suffering

through a long illness, a sibling who died in childhood, a friend diagnosed one week and dead the next. Sometimes they cry, and I comfort them. They apologize, but they don't have to. I find their stories strangely consoling. I begin to realize how many people carry within them the permanent imprint of someone who is no longer here, how many people leave an indelible mark after they are gone. I begin to see how people can live through the death of a loved one, never forgetting but still finding a way to go on.

I develop a routine of heading into San Francisco after I drop Matthew at school, working through lunch, and then leaving in time to beat the afternoon rush. I park the car in a lot near the BART station and ride the train in and out of the city. Because I travel off-hours, I almost always get a choice of seats. I select one as far from other people as I can and turn my face toward the window, black as midnight for most of the underground route. The train ride becomes my grieving time. With no one watching, no one worrying, no one caring what I do, I allow myself to feel the full weight of the sadness, the fear, the dread, the panic, and the yearning that I usually deny. The other passengers bury their faces in newspapers or nap; they don't notice the silent tears that slide down my face and splash on my coat. The thirty-minute ride becomes my private crying session, three days a week.

Today, I descend into the BART station to find it unusually crowded for midday. The video monitors announce that there is a delay somewhere down the line, causing a backup. When my train pulls in, I get a seat, but every other seat is filled, as well.

In the seat facing mine, a well-dressed woman about my age is looking at me as if she recognizes me. She doesn't look familiar, so I turn away, hoping to avoid conversation.

My tears flow involuntarily as I turn my face toward the window. I feel someone touch my hand. It is the woman sitting opposite me. She leans toward me and whispers, "Is there anything I can do?" Her expression is kind and intelligent.

"I'm okay," I say. "My husband died recently, and I get weepy sometimes."

"I thought so," she says. "I know how you feel. I lost my husband several years ago."

I look at her with sympathy but also with interest. "How did your husband die?"

"We were on a cruise," she says. "We were snorkeling—my husband, my daughter, and I. We were just swimming around, looking at the fish. Suddenly, my husband wasn't with us anymore. We swam around looking for him and then figured that he must have gone back to the ship. We don't really know what happened. He must have had a cramp or something. They found his body a few hours later."

"How terrible for you. And for your daughter."

"It's always roughest on the kids. They never completely get over it."

"Never?"

She shakes her head. "They get on with their lives, of course, much better than adults do. But when children lose a parent, they lose a part of themselves. They will always be searching for that missing piece."

We ride in silence for a moment, and then she says, "You have children." It is a statement rather than a question.

I nod. "Two boys."

"Have you gotten help for them?"

I sigh. "We went to a counselor for a while, but my younger son refused to talk and my older son said it was a waste of time."

"Find someone else. They need help, believe me, especially the one who refuses to talk."

"Any recommendations?"

"Do you have a piece of paper?"

I pull out my date book, open it to a blank page, and offer it to her with a pen. She scribbles a name and number and passes it back.

"This organization works specifically with kids who have problems. They have group therapy for kids with a terminally ill parent, kids who have been exposed to violence, and kids who have lost a parent. They do amazing things. They helped my daughter understand what she was feeling about her father's death, and she met other kids who were in the same situation, which was invaluable."

"Where are they located?" I ask.

The train is lurching to a stop. The woman gets up, slinging her purse over her shoulder. "They have a small building up in the Oakland hills," she says. "Call them soon. There's usually a waiting list." Then she wishes me luck and is gone.

"There is no doubt about it," Karin says firmly. "That woman was a transfiguration."

Karin and I are sitting in the aromatherapy room of the day spa, swaddled in white terry, still limp from being worked over by Karin's massage therapist. "What is a transfiguration?" I ask. After that massage, I'm perhaps more open-minded than I otherwise might be. I have no idea what she is talking about, but in conversations with Karin, I'm often in over my head.

"The woman you met on BART was actually Nick. He took a physical form in order to deliver a message."

"What was the message?"

"Didn't she give you a number to call to get help for Matthew?"

"That's the message? *That's* what he has to say to me?"

"He's obviously concerned about his son."

I unwrap the towel that loosely circles my neck and let it drop to the floor. The towel is infused with a eucalyptus scent that I had hoped would help ease my breathing, but instead it's starting to give me a headache.

"Why would Nick be getting involved now? And what about that three-day or three-week thing?"

Karin sighs and readjusts her lounge chair. "Three days is the time that a person has after death to achieve closure. But there are lots of cases where spirits linger around their loved ones for years, offering guidance and protection."

"So Nick has been watching over me all this time?" I don't believe this for a minute.

The attendant, a muscular woman, placid to the point of somnolence, glides noiselessly among the dozen lounge chairs arranged around the softly lit room. She tops off glasses of lemon ice water from the nearest of several pitchers that sit on corner tables, and she asks if she can refresh our towels. I'm trying to picture Nick hovering over me. Where was he when I poked myself in the eye and couldn't drive for a week? Or when I cracked my rib, which is still aching? I could have used his guidance with the furnace noises, with the sliding hillside, with the broken gutter. Where was he then? Why didn't he guide me away from finding Kathy's letter?

A thought occurs to me. "If the dead linger around their loved ones," I say to Karin, "then was Rachael hovering over Nick when I met him? Was she there the day we got married? Did she come with us on our honeymoon?"

"I don't think that the dead are interested in your sex life."

The attendant returns with a lavender towel. "Lavender is for soothing, calming," she breathes, tucking the freshly scented towel under my chin.

"That woman may not have been an apparition," Karin says thoughtfully.

"You thought the towel woman was Nick, too?" I ask, incredulous.

Unexpected Help

Karin gives me an exasperated look. "I'm talking about the woman on BART," she says. "It occurs to me that she might be a real person that Nick selected and guided into your path."

I start to ask why it doesn't occur to her that the woman I met on BART may have been just that: a woman I met on BART. But my headache is fading, and I'm finding that the warmth of the towels combined with the wafts of lavender are soothing and calming after all, and I've no interest in debating the issue any further.

"It doesn't really matter who the woman was," Karin says practically. "You should still call the number she gave you."

More Hoops to Jump Through

chapter thirty-eight

I call Jerry to get an adoption update. "I got a preliminary copy of the probation officer's report, and everything looks good," he says. "Does your son really have his own twenty-seven-inch TV, VCR, and computer in his room?"

"The TV and VCR are both old, and the computer is mostly for his homework," I say defensively.

"The report does say that your son seems very unspoiled," he says, trying to make up for it. "Anyway, the probation officer can finalize the report once he's heard back from all the jurisdictions you've lived in. Of course, we are not expecting anything to turn up."

"How long do you think it will take?"

"About another month," Jerry says, "maybe less, who knows? In the meantime, there is one other hoop we have to jump through. You will have to get three people to write letters in support of the adoption."

More Hoops to Jump Through

My stomach clenches. "I thought you said all I'd have to ask the Miners to do was sign the adoption request."

"These letters have to be written by people who are *not* related to Nikolaus or to you. You can pick anyone—teachers, coaches, Scouts leaders, and ministers tend to make good references. And, most important, they are used to writing letters."

"Can I just ask a neighbor or a friend?"

"That's fine, but be prepared to write the letters for them and then just have them sign at the bottom. Friends and neighbors may be eager to help, but you'll be surprised at how hard it is for most people to write a simple letter."

It turns out that Jerry is right. Despite enthusiastic responses to my request, it takes several phone calls and more than two months before I get three completed letters to the court.

Common Ground

chapter thirty-nine

When I call the number the woman on BART gave me, I find out that there is a six-month waiting list for the children's grief group. The woman on the phone is very apologetic. "We always have more people in need than we can handle," she says wearily.

But six weeks later, I receive a call. "A space for your son has become available. The session starts tonight. Can you make it?"

"We'll be there," I promise.

I don't exactly tell Matthew the whole truth about where we are going. "Just because you have to go to some dumb meeting, I don't see why I have to go," Matthew complains. "Why can't I just stay home with Nikolaus?"

"Nikolaus has homework," I say. I actually would make Nikolaus come, but the age limit is twelve. "Plus, other people in my meeting are bringing kids, too, so it might be fun."

He remains unconvinced. I'm not sure how he'll react when he figures out what this meeting is really about, but I figure that I'll cross that bridge later.

He sulks in the car and lags behind as we walk into the building. At least he doesn't make me drag him in. That always makes a bad first impression.

In the small lobby, there are three kids playing a game of tag under the watchful eyes of their mothers, who are sitting on a small bench nearby. "You can join in if you like," I whisper to Matthew. "No, thanks," he says firmly. More adults and children are arriving, and soon, a young woman comes out of the main door to greet us.

She passes around a sign-in sheet and introduces four volunteer counselors. Three are psychology students at a nearby university. The fourth is a man about my age, perhaps a bit older. The psychology students invite the kids to follow them to the "playroom." The man will meet with the adults in a separate room. "I'll just stick with you," Matthew says.

"You need to go with the kids. I have work to do." I am firm, unyielding.

One of the students takes Matthew's hand. Matthew lets himself be led away, although he drags his feet and shoots pleading looks at me until he is out of sight.

The adults gather in a large room off the foyer. The group consists of one man and six women, myself included. The man, Aaron, introduces himself as the facilitator. He is a volunteer, he lost his wife to cancer five years ago, he's been through training, whatever, whatever. I've heard this all before.

I expect we'll begin by telling our stories as we did in the other group, but I am wrong. Aaron starts by talking about the kids. "Tonight, the student counselors will be reading your kids a story about a little boy who feels one way inside but acts differently on the outside. Then they will make masks while the counselors encourage them to talk about the difference between how they look on the outside and how they are really feeling on the inside." I wonder if Matthew will participate or sit in the corner and sulk.

We do introduce ourselves, but our stories are kept short. Carolyn is a frazzled blond with two kids, a boy and a girl, seven and eight. Her husband died of cancer. Next is Kelly, a small, neatly dressed woman, whose husband also died of cancer. Kelly has a nine-year-old daughter. Abby is a tall, thin redhead with two girls, nine and eleven. Her husband died of a heart attack. Then there is Shirley, noticeably younger than the rest of us, who confuses everyone by announcing that she is "a newlywed." She rushes to explain, "I just buried my mother and father. They were like my son's parents. Of course, he has a new dad now." She wiggles her wedding ring at us and rambles on, "I was nineteen when I got pregnant, so Tommy and I have always lived with my parents. I inherited the house, of course, which is perfect with me being newly married and all. But of course Tommy still misses his Nonny and Pop Pop."

An uncomfortable minute passes, and it is obvious that we are all trying to digest this barrage of information while Shirley, oblivious, placidly admires the speck of diamond on her hand. Finally, Aaron says, "Let's talk about what you are expecting your kids to get out of the group." He turns to two women sitting side by side. "Carolyn and Kelly, your kids have been here before. Can you share some of your experiences?"

Carolyn and Kelly, it turns out, both had their kids in the Living with a Serious Illness group for several months. They moved their kids to the Coping with Grief group after their husbands died. Although their children were among the group I had seen playing tag in the lobby—laughing and pushing each other playfully—both women described their kids as withdrawn, listless, and angry.

"It sounds like you're describing my son," I say. "How do you cope with their behavior without punishing them more?" Carolyn and Kelly offer thoughtful suggestions, and Abby joins in with concerns and questions. For the first time, I feel like I'm with people who not only have the same problems as I do but are working on real solutions. Shirley listens but doesn't seem to have much to add. Aaron lets the conversation flow.

Two hours fly by. I'm surprised when I hear the kids pounding on the door, each one clutching a brightly colored mask, still wet with paint. Matthew's is black and blue. "Here, you hold it," he says, shoving it in my hands as he runs outside with the other kids, who are now tossing a Frisbee around a small, square lawn. If he is still mad at me for bringing him here, he seems to have forgotten about it, at least for the moment, as he vies for the attention of whichever kid is currently holding the Frisbee and dives to reach any throw that comes his way. But afterward, in the car, he gives terse answers to my careful questions.

"Did you read a story?" I ask.

"Yeah."

"Was it interesting?"

"Not really."

"Did you have fun making the mask?"

"Not really."

Still, I'm encouraged when I see him carry his mask into the house instead of leaving it in the back seat with his other forgotten toys.

Later, I find the mask face down in the garbage can.

—⚏—

Matthew complains loudly about going to the group the next week. "The kids are dumb," he says, "and they do boring stuff." I have to drag him into the car, and when we arrive at the small building, he refuses to budge.

"Fine with me," I finally say. "You can just sit here for two hours while I go inside to the meeting."

"Fine with me, too," he retorts. He emphatically crosses his arms, tucking his hands in his armpits and squeezing his chest so hard his face reddens.

Through the lobby's plate glass doors, I can see the back of his small head held high above the edge of the car's seat. I know he won't give me the satisfaction of turning around.

One of the women I met last week, Carolyn, is standing next to a small boy, watching as I leave the car with Matthew still inside. She turns to the little boy and says, "Russell, go ask that little boy sitting in the car if he wants to play Frisbee with you." Russell pauses a moment and then, deciding not to protest, trots reluctantly off. He knocks on the window of the car, and Matthew opens the door. Brief words are exchanged, and Matthew shrugs and gets out of the car. Together, the boys walk across the parking lot to the small front lawn.

"Thank you," I say to Carolyn.

"No problem," she says. "Actually, your son seems to be doing better than most," she tells me. "I had to physically drag my kids to the first few meetings."

"Did they do that thing where they pretend to collapse while they are still hanging on to your arm?" I ask. "Matthew does that to me almost every day. One of my arms is now two inches longer than the other."

Carolyn laughs in recognition.

The counselors are already rounding up the kids. Matthew pointedly ignores me as he and his new friend climb the stairs to the kids' meeting room.

The adults gather in the smaller room, and we sit in a circle like last week. Aaron tells us that the kids will be making collages out of magazine pictures. Shirley, the twentysomething newlywed, announces that she will be leaving the group early tonight. "My husband and I spent the day stripping the wall-paper in the front bedroom. I promised I'd be back early so we could finish the final coat tonight." She proudly displays the paint splatters that still cling to her hands and arms. "It's so nice to be able to fix the house the way that we want it now that . . ." her voice trails off, but it is perfectly clear that she was about to say "now that my parents are gone." She turns bright red and falls mercifully silent.

A half an hour later, the rest of us are in the middle of discussing whether it is appropriate to make our children visit their fathers' graves if they don't want to when Shirley sneaks out.

In the car on the way home, Matthew says, "You know that kid I was playing with? His dad died, too."

"Tonight, the kids will be talking about ways to remember and honor the person they lost," Aaron says, "while also not being afraid to change and move on with life."

Shirley is eager to jump in, and her words rush like a fast-moving stream. "My son is really adjusting well to all the changes. Of course, he has a new dad now. My husband is such a great guy. He and Tommy really get along great together." Shirley is oblivious to the gaping stares resulting from these remarks. She sits cross-legged, slightly rocking, her hair scraped up into two small pigtails that sprout from pink butterfly barrettes. She looks like she should be upstairs with the kids. "My husband has just made it so much easier for me and Tommy to get over my parents' death. I know I am so lucky to be married to such a great guy."

"Good for you." Carolyn's tone is neutral, but her sarcasm is clear, even to Shirley, whose high spirits deflate faster than a pricked balloon. "I miss my mom and dad so much," she suddenly wails. "When you lose your mom and dad like I did . . . Well, you just don't know how hard it is."

Carolyn stares at Shirley. "I think we might have a clue."

There is a palpable tension in the air. I would not be surprised if Shirley bursts into tears, or if Carolyn strikes her. Kelly's lips are pressed together so hard they are white, and Abby is busily studying her fingernails.

"Let's get back on the subject," Aaron says. "Let's talk about some of the things around us that remind us of our loved ones."

Shirley is anxious to make amends, to get back with the program. "We are living in my mom and dad's house, so that reminds me of them every day."

Aaron turns to Kelly. "How is your bonsai collection doing?"

Kelly shakes her head ruefully. "I'm afraid they are almost all dead," she says, then explains to the group, "My husband, Dan, was really into bonsai, and he loved working on them. After he died, I tried to take care of his plants because they reminded me of him. But I'm finding out that I don't have the time or the expertise to keep them alive." She takes in a long breath. "Frankly, I'll be glad when they're all gone. It's hard to watch them slowly turning brown and dying. And to tell you the truth, I never really liked bonsai all that much. I'd rather have something else to remember him by."

"I know exactly what you're saying," Abby says. "My husband collected wine. I now have cases and cases of wine—really fine, expensive wine—more than I'll ever be able to drink. I wish that we had opened more of it while Karl was still alive to enjoy it, but there's nothing I can do about that now. I put aside a few bottles for the girls to open on their wedding days, or when their children are born, or whatever. But the rest I'm just trying to use up. I'm pouring vintage wines into spaghetti sauce and beef stew."

"It's funny how the things that were most important to our husbands wind up being the most burdensome things to us," Carolyn observes. "For me, it was the house. We didn't have any money when we were first married, and so we bought a really small, junky house. Over the years, Eric rebuilt that house by hand. Since we didn't have the money to hire workers who knew what they were doing, the house was full of quirks that only Eric knew how to fix." She smiles at the memory and then turns serious. "Eric had a form of leukemia when he was a teenager, so he was never able to get life insurance. We had trouble getting basic health insurance. After he died, I had to sell the house right away to pay off the medical bills. It really killed me to sell that house, but staying there with all those memories, upkeep aside, would have been a slow death for me."

Kelly reaches over and hugs Carolyn. "You did the right thing to sell it."

"I had no choice," Carolyn says, wiping her eyes. "But there are easier things to keep than a house to remember Eric by."

"I'll have to sell my house, too," I say. "I've been delaying the sale until my older son finishes high school, but I think I've also kept it because that house is the one place on earth that I know my husband would come back to."

"Has he ever come back?" Abby asks. "In spirit, or his ghost, or whatever?"

"No," I say. "I've tried to reach him. But now I think my mother-in-law is right—when you're dead, that's it."

Shirley has been quiet, but now she says, "I loved that movie where Patrick Swayze comes back to help Demi Moore figure out who killed him."

Aaron says, "In real life, frankly, I've never seen any evidence of an afterlife communication."

Carolyn adds, "I'm so tired all the time, I think I could easily hallucinate that Eric is sending me a message. I haven't really slept well since Eric died."

"I think that Dan is somewhere, waiting for me," Kelly says, "but I hope he has a really long wait."

Moving Out

chapter forty

I know that sooner or later, I'll have to do something about Nick's clothes. I run my hand over the line of suits, the row of carefully pressed slacks, and the stacks of sweaters, and I think about Kelly's bonsai trees, Abby's wine collection, and Carolyn's house. I think about the careful tailoring of the suits, the custom-made dress shirts, the pants hemmed at just the right length—all designed to the taste and fit and preferences of one specific individual.

Nick's clothes seemed to be a big concern of everyone's in the days after the funeral. It was an easy thing for other people to focus on, but the last thing I wanted to think about. Several people volunteered to help clean out his closet, but I put them off. "There will be plenty of time for that," I'd say. "There are so many more important things to do now."

Until now, I've been in no hurry to decide what to do with Nick's clothes. Until now, they've helped me believe in the fantasy that Nick might actually not be gone forever. I know that when his clothes are gone, half of the closet, half of my life, will be empty.

Suddenly, I see how pathetic it is to keep them. Kelly tends the bonsai, waiting and hoping for each to die so that she will be free of them. Abby works her way through endless cases of wine, one glass at a time. I have the opportunity to make a clean break.

Tom excuses my failure to purge the clothes by suggesting that I might be saving some of them for the boys. I can't picture them thanking me for that. Who would want to inherit a wardrobe of half-worn clothes that probably won't fit?

"When my dad retired, he gave all his suits and things to a job-training program in San Francisco," Melanie had mentioned several weeks ago. "I have their number if you want it."

I call the number and connect with a woman who seems very excited about the possibility of getting a dozen suits, shoes, and accessories. "Can you possibly bring them this week?" she asks. "We have several men about to complete our program who could use them." I set a time to deliver them the next day.

I decide to pack Nick's suits first. One by one, I transfer them off the heavy cedar hangers and onto cheap plastic ones. I've already done a thorough search of all Nick's pockets. Now I let my hands linger one last time over the soft wool, the silk linings, the labels embroidered with his name. I carry them downstairs in armfuls and lay them carefully in the trunk of the car.

The shirts are next. They hang on flimsy, white wire hangers, organized by color. Crisp, white, starched collared shirts with faint white initials embroidered on the cuffs give way to whites with thin stripes of red, blue, or black, then the solid light blues and pale pinks. Then come the odd colors and styles: light and dark blue denim, black broadcloth, collarless linen and khaki, and polos and other knits. I save a few that Nikolaus or I might wear and carry the rest out to the car.

I fill two large plastic garbage bags with sweaters and sweat-shirts and an additional one with T-shirts. The trunk is full, and I have to put the bag of pajamas, socks, and shoes on the back seat. I haven't even tackled the dresser yet, but Nick's side of the closet is now mostly empty, and the car is packed.

I lean against the closed car door and then slide down it until I'm sitting on the concrete garage floor. I hug my knees to my chest. I don't notice how much time passes. I don't notice Nikolaus walking up the driveway from school until he is right next to me. "Are you crying?" he asks. "What happened?"

"I moved Papa out of the house," I say, wiping away the tears that I now feel burning on my cheeks. "His clothes, his shoes, everything . . ." I motion to the trunk.

He pats my back. "Don't cry. If you want, we can bring it all back in. I'll help you."

Yes, I think. *Yes. Let's bring it all back in. We don't have to do this. I'll call the job-training lady and tell her to forget it. I'll hang everything back up. Nikolaus will help me.*

"Thanks," I say, using the bottom of my shirt to dry my face, "but no. It needs to be done, and I'm halfway there. If we stop now, we'll just have to go through it all again later."

I think about the empty side of the closet. I think about facing it every day. "There is something you *can* help me with, though," I say to Nikolaus. Together, we find the box of ski clothes in the storage area under the house. We unfold the bibs, the big puffy jackets, the ski pants. We bring them upstairs and put them on the cedar hangers. By dinnertime, Nick's side of the closet is no longer empty.

Divorce Is Different

chapter forty-one

"I heard about a great single parents' group," Annemarie says. "It's time you got out a little bit. Why don't you come with me to check it out?"

I put her off for several weeks before I reluctantly agree to go. The group meets in the basement of a local church on Wednesday nights. Before we leave, Annemarie insists that I put on some makeup. "At least do your eyes up," she insists, and it seems easier to comply than argue, so I do.

The meeting has already started when we take our seats. Of the twenty or so people in the circle, about half are men. "Some of the guys are cute," Annemarie whispers, "and they're all available."

Unlike the grief group, we are not asked to introduce ourselves. The moderator, a pleasant, gray-haired woman, is in the midst of introducing tonight's topic, which is also posted on a large whiteboard that hangs against one wall. The topic, spelled out in large, black letters, is "Disappointment." "Think about the topic, and just shout out anything that comes to mind," the moderator says.

"I'm disappointed that my marriage failed," says one woman. Under "Disappointment," the moderator writes "Failed marriage."

"I'm disappointed that my husband didn't call our son on his birthday," says another. The moderator writes "Ex doesn't keep promises."

"My custody arrangement is really disappointing," a man adds. "In fact, it sucks." The moderator writes "Custody of children."

The litany of disappointments continues for about fifteen minutes, and then the moderator suggests taking a break. "Take five minutes to grab a cup of coffee or a soft drink from the back of the room, and then let's come back and work on some solutions," she says.

"Do you want something to drink?" I ask Annemarie. Almost everyone else is already heading back to the refreshment table.

"Of course," she says, eyes sparkling as she surveys the back of the room. "Let's go mingle." She grabs my arm, leaving me no choice but to follow her. As we make our way to the coffeepot, I can hear snatches of various conversations.

"My lawyer advised me to write *everything* down. Believe me, I have quite a list going."

"Which judge ruled on your settlement? I'm in court next week, but maybe I'll try to postpone."

"Are you throwing yourself a birthday party? Let me give you my new number."

Annemarie darts over to talk with the man who was complaining about his custody arrangements.

A voice behind me asks, "Have you been divorced long?" and it takes me a moment to realize that the question is directed at me. I turn to face a small, dark man in a leather jacket. I'm not sure how to answer his question; I just shrug.

"Leave her alone, John," a woman behind him says, and then, in a stage whisper to me, she adds, "He's always the first one to hit on newcomers."

I nod, pretending to be too busy pouring my coffee and stirring in the powdered cream to answer. I force a smile as I pick up my cup and retreat back to my seat.

Annemarie comes back just before the session starts up again. "Two guys asked for my phone number," she whispers, excited. "And the guy in the blue sweater over there was asking me about you."

The guy Annemarie points out is smiling broadly at us. He waves, and Annemarie waves back. There is no way I'm ready for this. I've made a big mistake coming here. I can't wait to be back in my own car, and in my own house. I stare down into my coffee and wait for the session to end.

Back to Life

chapter forty-two

When Matthew and I arrive at the kids' group the next week, Carolyn and Kelly are standing on the lawn, watching the kids play tag.

"I knew she wouldn't last," Carolyn is saying as I walk up.

"Did something happen?" I ask.

"Shirley dropped out," Kelly tells me, "or, more likely, they asked her to leave."

"They can do that?" This thought had never crossed my mind.

Carolyn nodded. "Their waiting list is so long that they can't keep a child in the group who they either can't help or who doesn't really need their help. I think Shirley's son probably fell into the latter category."

Tonight, for the first time, Matthew did not fight me about coming to the group. Now, as I watch him chasing the other kids around on the lawn, I believe it's one of the first times I've heard him laugh in months. Last week, the children's counselor told me that Matthew seldom talked in the group. "Some kids never talk," he reassured me, "but I can tell that Matthew is listening to the other kids, and that's helping him understand what he is feeling."

"Remember the newlyweds in the last session?" Kelly asks. Carolyn nods and laughs, then tells me the story. "Last session, there was a kid whose dad had died. His parents were divorced, and the mother came to a few meetings with her new husband. They were all over each other—sitting on each other's laps, tickling, playing kissy face. It was embarrassing. And neither of them had one nice thing to say about the poor kid's real dad. They were gone in two weeks. I felt sorry for the kid. I think they were referred to family counseling."

"Still, it seems kind of harsh to kick people out," I say.

"No one is allowed to stay for more than two eight-week sessions," Kelly informs me. "At the end of the first session, they counsel you on your child's progress, and you can decide whether to continue in the group or not. Carolyn and I are out after this session ends, since this is our second."

"Do you think your kids will be ready to leave?" I ask them.

Carolyn says, "I think they are ready to move on, but I'm not sure I am. You are the only people I've found who really understand what I'm going through. I'll miss that."

—◊—

Matthew and I arrive for the last session with our just-baked cupcakes. The group is meeting early tonight for a potluck picnic. Carolyn and Kelly are teary-eyed at the thought of leaving the group. "We'll keep in touch," we all promise, knowing as we say it that, as single mothers, most of us with full-time jobs, it is unlikely that we will find the time to get together very often.

After we eat the chicken wings, baked beans, and green salad, the kids and their counselors head upstairs with their cupcakes while the adults linger on the lawn, enjoying the unseasonably warm evening and watching the sun set over distant trees.

"The only reason I became a counselor," Aaron says, mostly joking, "is so that I wouldn't have to leave the group."

"Carolyn and I are thinking of joining that single parents' group Gloria enjoyed so much," Kelly says mischievously. "I bet we'll both be remarried by the time the rest of you finish the next session."

"I don't think I want to remarry," Carolyn protests, only half kidding now. "I'm getting used to being on my own."

"I think remarriage would be hard on my kids," Abby says. "I'm not sure they'll ever be ready to accept someone in their father's place."

"There's a lot about marriage I miss," Kelly says wistfully. "I miss having dinner with another adult, reading the Sunday paper together. . . ."

"I miss having someone to take out the garbage and mow the lawn," Abby confesses. "Now I do all the chores myself."

"And then there's sex," Carolyn adds.

Kelly shudders. "The thought of undressing in front of someone new may keep me single forever."

"You may not feel that way forever," Aaron responds. Over the past weeks, we've come to view him as one of the girls, and he's not at all uncomfortable jumping into this conversation. "I read somewhere that on average, widows remarry within five years of their husbands' deaths. Widowers generally remarry within a year or two."

"That's because men can't last too long on their own," Carolyn points out.

"Or because women won't leave them alone," Kelly says. "My husband, Dan, was a builder. There were lots of times when his female clients made it very clear that they were interested in more than his carpentry skills."

"How did you feel about that?" I ask.

Kelly shrugs. "It's par for the course. Dan was successful in business because he was a good listener. Everything he built was customized, and he made his clients feel like they were working together to build something really special. Some of his female clients misunderstood the partnership and tried to take it a bit too far."

"Just for the record, Aaron," Carolyn says, in an attempt to lighten the mood, "none of us are after you."

"I once found a love note written to my husband by a woman he worked with," I divulge. I have not shared this with anyone except my therapist since that day with Annemarie and Janine, but being able to admit it out loud feels good.

"Only once?" Abby asks sarcastically. "I have a whole collection of them. There was an endless series of twentysomething women who worked for my husband, and they were always writing him love notes." Her eyes flutter skyward as she imitates a young girl's singsong voice, "Dear Karl, you are so wonderful. I know we are destined to spend the rest of our lives together." I chuckle along with everyone else, but inside, I feel an uncomfortable twinge of recognition.

"I mostly felt sorry for them, really," Abby says. "It can be hard to find a man who's willing to make a commitment. When you are single and in your twenties moving toward thirty, you think it will never happen. They looked at Karl and saw a man who had a successful business, a home, and a family. And that's just the kind of man they want. What they don't realize is that it's like reaching for a reflection in a pond. The minute you grab it, not only is it gone, but you're the one who has destroyed it."

"Didn't you ever feel that your marriage was threatened by all that attention?" I ask.

"Not really. I'm sure that on some level, the attention was an ego boost for Karl," she says, nodding toward Aaron, "but he had to maintain a professional relationship with those women. I'm not saying he didn't flirt a bit from time to time, but I know he would never have crossed the line. If he had, he would have been jeopardizing everything that was important to him—his job, our marriage, his relationship with his kids."

This sounds familiar. It is the same conclusion I came to in Ryan's office when we first talked about the letter. I had a good husband, a good marriage. No one could take that away from me then, and certainly no one is going to take that away from me now.

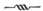

There is a break of a few weeks before the next group session begins. Matthew doesn't enthusiastically agree to rejoin the group, but he doesn't need a great deal of coaxing, either. Three new women are at the first meeting, replacing Carolyn, Kelly, and Shirley. Two are graduates from the Living with Illness group, and the other's husband recently died in a car accident.

The three new widows all have the hollow-eyed, shell-shocked expression that has now disappeared from my own face. They walk more slowly than I do, talk more softly, fall more easily into periods of silence. Their downcast eyes focus on some internal picture, in turns exquisite and terrifying. They move as if in a dream, apart from others, in some private universe.

I knew exactly where they are. I myself have only recently returned.

PART 3 The Beginning

Milestones

chapter forty-three

There are certain days that will always have an edge of sadness for us.

Nick died in February, so by the time Thanksgiving and Christmas come around, we have already made our way through a whole calendar of special days. Mother's Day. Father's Day. The kids' birthdays. Our wedding anniversary. My birthday. Nick's birthday. I brace myself for each occasion, praying that the day won't be defined by sorrow and intense emotions, grateful just to get through it unscathed.

As Christmas draws near, I begin to notice that everywhere we go, the smiles on people's faces slowly fade when they greet us. I watch them turn and hug their husbands, their fathers, their children just a little tighter. They look at us and see sorrow. We are a shadow of what could happen, a trigger that reminds them to be thankful for everything they still have. I feel like Tiny Tim, sitting in church so that others may see us and count their blessings.

It seems important to decorate the house, to trim the tree, to have piles of presents—to prove that we are normal. We have enough lights to outline the entire house. Despite my objections, Nick used to insist on climbing to the top of the house, three stories up, to hang our lights. I won't even go to the second story and will not allow Nikolaus to do it, either. I don't want him to do the foolhardy things that his father did. I want to keep him safe. Despite loud objections from Matthew, we hang four strings of lights around the porch and use a few more to outline the garage door. In years past, when Nick had the house ablaze with lights, I remember it seemed like a safe haven, shining out in the dark night. Now, with its few paltry strands of light, the house looks to me like a great, dark ship that's getting ready to sail away to some unseen destination.

The boys refuse to compromise on the tree. It has to be at least an eight-footer. Nick could climb the front stairs with a ten-foot tree hoisted on his shoulder. This year, it takes Nikolaus and me over an hour to wrestle our smaller specimen into the living room, leaving a trail of water and needles tracing our path across the driveway, up the front steps, and through the hall.

"Why didn't you just have the tree delivered?" Janine asks, surveying the scratches that still adorn my arms a week afterward. It never occurred to me. We always brought the tree home ourselves. But I am not afraid of change. We are free to start new traditions.

We invite the Miners to join us for Christmas dinner, but only Rob Miner comes. Nikolaus is disappointed; I try not to show my relief. Rob brings presents for both boys. Ruth and Robyn send three or four presents each for Nikolaus—candy, a video game, a radio for his room, a remote control car. They send Matthew a sweater that doesn't fit. It doesn't matter. Big boxes of presents arrive from my family. I resisted my mother's attempts to get us to go east for the holidays—I think it's important that Nikolaus, Matthew, Elisabeth, and I are home together. I make a big pot of soup, and we spend the day in sweatpants watching a James Bond movie marathon on TV. It's a perfect day.

Almost everyone we know stops by at some point during the holiday week to bring "a little something for the kids." Even Matthew quickly figures it out. "Is everyone giving us presents just because Papa died?" he asks me.

Our toughest day comes well after Christmas. Our toughest day is February 7, the anniversary of the day Nick died. It's a day that didn't have any significance while Nick was still with us, but now it looms on the calendar like a huge, black shadow. It is not a day I particularly want to remember, but it seems appropriate to do something to honor his memory.

Nick died on a Saturday, so the first anniversary of his death falls on a Sunday. Elisabeth and the boys and I go to church in the morning and then to the cemetery. We stand in a small circle around Nick's grave. I read a poem by e. e. cummings.

when by now and tree by leaf
she laughed his joy she cried his grief
bird by snow and stir by still
anyone's any was all to her

We tie a bouquet of silk roses on his headstone, the one that I finally ordered for him. It is made of the same kind of granite that Nick and I had picked out for our kitchen. There is a picture of Nick that I took on our honeymoon, along with his name, his birthday, and the day he died. There is enough room underneath to add my name and my dates, maybe, someday, a long time from now. On the base of the stone, I had them carve an inscription:

Milestones

Death is a horizon, no more than the limits of our sight.
You live in our hearts forever, beloved.

I know now that it is foolish to think that the dead can communicate with the living. The dead live on, but only in the hearts and minds of those they loved, those who loved them, those whose lives they touched. The rock we throw into the pond of life continues to ripple after we die, some ripples lasting longer and stronger than others, but all fading inevitably with time.

"We can't see Papa anymore," I tell Matthew, "but we will never forget him."

"Nicky, we sure miss you," Elisabeth says, touching the picture.

It's been a long, hard year, one that I wouldn't wish on anyone. But we've come through it, and we've survived.

Leaving
Memories
Behind

chapter forty-four

The summer before Nikolaus will graduate from high school, I begin to look for a smaller house. It seems like it should take a long time to find something that we won't feel bad about moving into. A year is barely enough to get used to the idea of moving.

I meet with a local real estate agent who comes highly recommended, and I lay out a list of nonnegotiable terms: Four bedrooms—one for me, one for Matthew, one to use as an office and guest room, and one for Nikolaus to come home to. No stairs for Elisabeth to climb. A big backyard with grass for Matthew. A feeling of privacy but with no acreage to maintain. Something that doesn't need a lot of work or upkeep. And within the price range specified by the financial advisor, which would allow me to realize a reasonable retirement and a comfortable old age.

I am dismayed when the first house the agent shows me meets all of my criteria. I was hoping for a longer search process.

But the house is neat and tidy, and it has an updated kitchen and a manageable yard. Before I finalize the offer, I bring the boys over to see it. They give their grudging approval.

"Can we still keep our real house?" Matthew asks.

Now that we know where we are moving, it's time to begin in earnest the process of letting the other house go.

We work to get it ready for sale. First, the real estate agent brings in a decorator to stage the house. She insists that we get rid of half the furniture, hangs rented paintings on the walls, and puts huge, fake trees in the living room. Dozens of throw pillows are arranged in careful groups on the couches and the beds, and more are scattered outside on the decks.

"We want the house to look comfortable," the decorator says.

"With all these pillows, there's no place to sit down," Matthew complains.

They ask us to pack away all family photos. "Prospective buyers might feel they are displacing you," the real estate agent explains.

"They *are* displacing us," I say.

"We're not being displaced," Nikolaus clarifies. "We are being invaded."

The decorator hides our toaster and our coffeemaker, artfully arranges wine glasses next to the bathtub, and ties bows around all the towels. It is virtually impossible for us to live in the house. The kids and I retreat to the new house, which holds the furniture that's been banished by the decorator and supplemented by lawn furniture.

Within a week, the agent has three offers, all at asking price or above.

The morning I'm to review the offers, I drop the kids off at school and then drive over to the house that I never thought I would sell. Seeing the realtor's sign standing at the end of the driveway feels like a nightmare. The irises and daffodils Nick and I planted are in full bloom, creating soft washes of purple and yellow around the decks. Dew sparkles across the newly laid lawn, and as I climb the hill, the weeds make a familiar *swish* on my legs.

At the top, I take a long, last look at the redwoods, the rocks, the rosemary. I gaze down on the outline of the house and think of everything that happened to me here. I arrived as a bride here and became a mother here—first to Nikolaus and then again, later, when we brought Matthew home. This house would forever hold the memories of losing Nick, of burying my husband. I sit in the grass and wait. The sun grows warmer, the wind rustles the trees, and still I wait. "This is your last chance, Nick," I say aloud. "Speak now, or forever hold your peace."

By noon, I am in the realtor's office. The offer I accept is several thousand dollars over our asking price and is accompanied by a picture of a family—a mom, a dad, and two red-haired kids—along with a handwritten note describing how much they like the house.

In the first few months after we move, I dream about the house often. Sometimes in my dreams, the new family is there, playing in the yard or having drinks on the deck. Sometimes I'm alone inside the house, wandering through the rooms. I wake up abruptly, disoriented, in a bedroom that takes me a moment to recognize as mine.

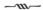

Several months after they move in, the new family invites us back to the house for dinner. "I hope you don't mind that we made some changes in the house," the wife calls from the kitchen as her husband hangs up our coats.

"I hope you don't mind that we cashed your check," Nikolaus mutters too softly, I hope, for them to hear him.

The kids play video games in the family room while the

adults take me on a tour. The house has changed very little, but still, it doesn't feel like the same place at all. The wallpaper in the dining room is gone. The kids' rooms are repainted. They invite me to look at the plans they are drawing up for a new deck. I follow them through the rooms, disoriented—as if some internal radar system has jammed. The beds are on the wrong sides of the rooms, the hall table is gone, and the couch is facing the fireplace instead of the windows. A huge painting hangs in the foyer where the mirror used to be.

Anyone would say that they decorated the house beautifully. But to me, walking through its rooms, it feels like a crazy house, where everything is slightly off kilter in a way that leaves you feeling breathless and dizzy. I know that the place I thought of as home no longer exists. After tonight, I know I will never dream about the house again.

Breaking
Family Ties

chapter forty-five

Nikolaus's adoption is finalized just three weeks before his eighteenth birthday. Rob Miner comes to court with us to witness the final decree. The juvenile court sets aside a special day each month to hear adoption cases, and the courtroom is filled with kids and their prospective moms and dads, many dressed in Sunday best, some holding balloons and brightly colored packages. There is a feeling of expectation and excitement as each family group is called into the judge's chambers to sign the final papers.

There is also the feeling that lives are being changed. But we are different. We undertook the legal process so that our lives would *not* change, so that we could remain as we had been all along. When the judge hands us our final papers, I feel mostly relieved.

A few weeks after the adoption is finalized, Nikolaus has dinner with Robyn and Jeff. When he comes home, he seems upset.

"Aunt Robyn told me some things about you," he says slowly, "and about Papa. I want to ask you if they're true."

I'm baffled. "Things about me and Papa? Like what?"

Nikolaus hesitates, and then he says, "She said that Papa didn't do a good job of taking care of my mother, you know, when she was sick."

The sad look on Nikolaus's face makes my heart ache. I'm not sure how to reassure him. I think for a moment, then say, "Your mother was very sick, and she was sick for a long time. Many people have said that Papa did a great job taking care of her. Your grandfather even said so at Papa's funeral. I can't tell you what happened or didn't happen, because I didn't know Papa then. But knowing the kind of man that your father was, I'm sure that he did everything he could for your mother."

Instead of being reassured by my words, Nikolaus looks away from me, embarrassed. Then he says, "She also said that you and Papa knew each other while my mother was still alive."

The full meaning of his words doesn't hit me right away. "I'm not sure what you mean."

"I mean Aunt Robyn says that you and Papa got together before my mother died," he says, miserable, but needing to know. "She says that Papa didn't take care of my mother because he was too busy fooling around with you."

His words sting as if I've been shot by a million needles. I feel angry, betrayed. I know that Robyn doesn't like me, but why would she make up such a story? At the same time, I feel an overwhelming sadness for Nikolaus. The story has been designed to hurt him in the worst way possible. Not only does it shake his trust in me, but worse, it denigrates his father, the man he most admired, the man he most loved.

It takes me a moment to organize my thoughts. I'm so furious with Robyn I can hardly see straight, but I have to be calm, so that Nikolaus will know the truth.

"That's not true," I say, trying to keep my voice from shaking, "That's the worst lie I have ever heard. Your mother had been gone for at least six months when I met Papa. I sat next to him on a plane. You've heard the story a million times."

"Aunt Robyn says it's not true," Nikolaus says miserably.

I feel bile rising in my throat. I swallow hard. "Why would she say that?"

"I don't know." I can see that this is tearing Nikolaus apart. "That's why I had to ask you if it was true."

I look him straight in the eye. "No, it is not true."

I search my brain for something I can use to prove my case. "Call Papa's friend Glenn. He knew Papa when your mother was alive. Ask him. Ask him what kind of man your father was." What I don't say is: *And find out what kind of person your Aunt Robyn is for telling such a story.*

Nikolaus looks downcast. "I believe you," he says.

"You don't have to believe me," I say. "Call Glenn. He has nothing to lose by telling you the truth."

Nikolaus doesn't call Glenn right away. But when he does finally reach out to him, Glenn tells him what I had told him: Nick and I met about six months after Rachael died. Nick and Glenn had lunch together the day after we met, and Nick excitedly told Glenn everything he knew about me. When Rachael was alive, Nick was too busy caring for a sick wife and a child to have the time or energy for an affair.

I've spent a lot of time thinking about why Robyn said these things about me to Nikolaus. Does she really believe them? Suddenly, I understand why she has always disliked me. Maybe this was all based on a misunderstanding. But why didn't she confront me years ago so that the truth could have come out? Or did she just make up this preposterous story? And why did she lay all of this on Nikolaus? And why now?

When Rob Miner finds out what his sister said, he takes it

upon himself to discuss it with Nikolaus. He calls me later and apologizes on Robyn's behalf.

I don't tell Nikolaus that he can't see Robyn anymore. He is eighteen now and old enough to make his own decisions. But one thing is clear to me—I don't want to have anything to do with her.

Strength in
Crisis

chapter forty-six

Elisabeth wants to go back to Germany to see her sister. I've never been to Europe, and Matthew, almost ten years old now, is mature enough to be able to appreciate and remember the trip. So we buy tickets and pack our bags.

We fly into Frankfurt in early July and spend several days adjusting to the time difference and settling Elisabeth with her sister in a small town in the Pflaz region. The kids and I then take a train to Amsterdam and meet up with an American tour group with which we will spend the next three weeks. There are twenty-five people on the tour. Among us are a few young couples, a few older couples, two or three single travelers, and a few families of various types—two sets of mom, dad, and kids; a father with his two daughters; a retired secretary with her adult daughter; and a plastic surgeon with her two teenage daughters.

We quickly settle into a routine. The bus takes us to a new

city every two or three days. We hit major cities—Amsterdam, Rome, Florence, Venice—as well as smaller ones, including an alpine village in Switzerland, a seaside town in northern Italy, and a small Austrian town. The routine is always the same. We settle into our hotel, usually a small bed-and-breakfast, often run by a local family. The couple that acts as our guide schedules a short orientation to the city for anyone who wants it. They give us some background on the city and its attractions, provide tips on transportation and restaurants, and arrange for tickets to major museums and other sites. Then we are on our own to explore.

An easy friendship develops among our group. Nikolaus immediately makes friends with several of the teenage girls, and since two of them are sisters traveling with their mother, our two families explore together. A young husband on his honeymoon asks Nikolaus to join him in climbing various towers and domes when his wife goes shopping. There are several single women on the tour—two teachers, the retired secretary, and the plastic surgeon. They seem to enjoy being included in our family group, and I welcome their company.

After three weeks of travel, the tour winds up in Paris on the night before Matthew's tenth birthday. Our guides make arrangements for a farewell dinner at a small, quaint restaurant, and everyone has a great time. The wine flows freely, and after dinner, we drift into a local café, reluctant to have the night, and the tour, end. I had promised Matthew a trip to Euro Disney the next day for his birthday, so we are the first to return to the hotel. Nikolaus stays with the group, enjoying his last night with his new friends.

At six the next morning, we are awakened by screaming. Marilyn, a woman who had been traveling with her thirty-something daughter, is in the hall shouting, "Help me! Help me! Please, somebody!"

Her room is next to ours, and I rush out to see what's wrong. She is hysterical. "It's my daughter! I can't wake her up! Help me, somebody, please!"

The door to their room is ajar, and I run inside. Her daughter is lying on the bed face up, her eyes closed. Her skin is a very pale blue. When I shake her, her arm is cold as a stone. There's no doubt. She's dead.

The plastic surgeon in our group comes in, takes the daughter's pulse, and shakes her head. The retired fireman attempts CPR. The woman's mother shrinks into one corner of the room and sobs.

The paramedics arrive and clear everyone out of the room. I take the sobbing mother back into our room and ask Nikolaus and Matthew to go down to the lobby and fetch her a cup of tea. By the time they return, Marilyn is self-possessed but hollow eyed. I hold her hand and offer small sips of tea. She tells me that her daughter was a diabetic, and Nikolaus runs to relay this information to the paramedics.

The Paris police arrive. I help translate their questions using what little high school French I remember. Where does the dead woman live? Who was she with last night? What time did she return to the hotel?

By now it's mid-morning, and the people in our group are getting anxious to be on their way. The tour is over. Some people are staying on in Paris, while others are heading for other cities or for home. The police are reluctant to let anyone leave until they finish their investigation, but as it is becoming increasingly apparent that the woman's death is related to her diabetes, they take everyone's names and addresses and let us go.

The kids and I had planned to sightsee in Paris for a few more days, but we had made arrangements to stay at a different hotel. The police ask Marilyn to come with them to the American embassy. The surgeon agrees to accompany her, while I take the surgeon's two daughters and my sons to our new hotel. I get the kids something to eat and arrange a room for the grieving mother so she won't have to spend another night in the hotel where her daughter died. Everyone else on the tour, all these people we spent weeks with on the road, including the tour guides, say quick goodbyes and leave.

During the days that follow, I have the strong feeling that I have been placed somewhere that I need to be. Marilyn stays in the hotel room next to us for three or four more days. I help her call her children and ex-husband back in the United States to let them know what happened. Marilyn and I take a cab across Paris to meet with the funeral director and make arrangements for cremation and shipment of the remains. I help her go through her daughter's suitcase and decide what to leave in Paris and what to take back home. I arrange with the hotel concierge to take away the things Marilyn doesn't want to keep. The kids and I make sure Marilyn eats, we help her change her travel arrangements, and, when everything is finished, we ride with her to the airport, where she catches her flight home.

During the whole process, I feel sad for this mother and her daughter. But what I also feel, probably for the first time since Nick's death, is totally competent to handle the situation I am in. It makes me realize that when death happens, I know what to do. I watched the people around us shrink away from the proximity of death, afraid of not knowing what to say, afraid of a display of emotion, afraid of facing the possibility of their own mortality. For me and my sons, death is not scary. It's not unfamiliar. It's not extraordinary. It's just something that happens. And it is something that we know how to help someone get through.

Moving On

chapter forty-seven

People say that God only gives you as much as you can handle. I think you have no choice but to play the hand you are dealt.

It has been three years now since Nick died.

We've grown accustomed to Nick's absence. He has now missed three Thanksgivings, three Christmases, and dozens of birthday celebrations, Scouts ceremonies, and school performances. He will miss many more holidays, graduations, and weddings. We will carry him with us to each of these occasions as a little ache in our hearts.

Nikolaus graduated from high school last spring. Elisabeth, Matthew, Tom, and I sat high in the bleachers, watching the progression of tiny specks in blue robes cross the football field to receive diplomas. None of us spoke Nick's name that night, but there was no need. He was in our thoughts.

Ruth and LeRoy Miner came to the graduation, but they sat apart from us. We didn't speak.

Moving On

Nikolaus is now finding his way through college. He's more worried about establishing his own life than about protecting me, which is as it should be. I know there are times when he hears his father's voice in his head guiding him, cheering him, nagging him. I hear my mother's voice in the same way, though she is still alive.

Slowly, over time, Matthew stopped running from memories of his father and started asking questions. Was Papa good at baseball? What was his favorite TV show? What was his favorite color? He combines my answers with his own distant memories. He is searching to form a picture of the man his father was and the kind of man he wants to become. It is a search that Matthew will never complete, no matter how long he lives.

Even my own memories of Nick are becoming less distinct. He belongs to another time, as irretrievable as the sweet-faced baby that Matthew used to be or the small, awkward boy that Nikolaus once was. I'm back at work, and I've taken on new clients. I frequently have friends over for dinner. I have season tickets to the local theater. My life has grown around the wound of Nick's death, the scars not visible but still felt.

On my last birthday, I decided to give myself a present. A local bookstore advertised a weekend writing seminar. The teacher was a nationally known writer whose work I admired. I signed myself up. Elisabeth came over to watch the boys. Saturday night, I returned to folded laundry, well-fed kids, and an immaculate house. On Sunday night, I brought home a huge ice cream cake, and we stuck candles in it and sang. When I blew out the candles, I wished that all my birthdays would turn out so well.

It felt very much like a beginning.

What I've Learned

appendix

People sometimes compare healing from grief to healing from a wound, but in reality, that's not how it works. A wound heals slowly over time, getting a little bit better each day. Grief is not like that. Grief is like having a deep, gaping hole in your gut that makes it impossible to think, to eat, to breathe. After a while, you learn to cover it up and pretend nothing has happened, but the hole is still there. Eventually, the hole gets smaller, easier to manage, easier to hide. But it's always there.

There are lots of things I've learned about grief, about being a widow.

Funerals are very important.

When a loved one dies, it is important to come together and honor his or her life. I'm not suggesting that you spend every cent you have on an elaborate funeral, but don't just delegate the planning of the service to your priest, minister, or funeral director. Ask for input from the people who knew your loved one best. Make a slide show of family pictures. Play music that has special meaning. Ask friends and relatives to share their memories, but also ask coworkers, neighbors, or anyone else with a story that sheds light on all the varied facets of the person's life. I admit that I obsessed over the limos at Nick's funeral (and the flowers and the food), but that's not what makes a funeral satisfying. I've never left a funeral thinking, *What a great coffin!* Or, *Did you see those flowers?* The most meaningful funerals are those I've left feeling that I'd had that one last chance to get to know that person better.

Everyone will want you to get over it fast. You won't.

After the funeral is over, everyone will get back to their own lives—except you.

Everyone else will pick up where they left off. They'll return to their jobs, their families, their joys, their problems, their favorite restaurants. For them, pretty much nothing will have changed.

For you, everything will have changed. If you were busy taking care of a sick husband, suddenly you'll find yourself with unwelcome time on your hands. If you have children, you may find yourself overwhelmed with the responsibility of suddenly being a single parent. If you and your husband were inseparable, you now find yourself very alone.

Nothing will taste, feel, sound, or look the same to you. You'll have to find new ways to cope with everyday life. You'll have to relearn how to sleep, how to eat dinner, how to dress. It will take months before you even begin to feel comfortable in your own life. Then something happens—an illness, your car breaks down, it's Christmas—and suddenly you'll feel lost again.

No one will understand this. You won't be able to explain it. If you are close to someone who has lost a spouse, please, please, be patient with that person. He or she really doesn't know when it will end.

Grief is not a road, it's a roller coaster.

In the beginning, you'll have some really, really bad days. Then, suddenly, you'll have a morning or an afternoon where you'll feel almost normal. You'll think, *I'm better now. I'm getting over it.* But that's when grief swings back and kicks you in the head.

Eventually, you'll be able to string together more and more good days. But the bad days will still happen. One day you feel great, the next day you find yourself sobbing on the subway. Anything can trigger a bad day—a birthday, an anniversary, a song, garbage pickup day. Then suddenly you'll realize you haven't had a bad day in a week. That's when you know that you'll survive.

Grieving is physically hard.

Grieving creates a physical state that equates being hit repeatedly by a thirty-pound rock. Your bones ache. Your stomach hurts. You can't breathe. You shake. You feel nauseous. You can't concentrate. Your short-term memory is shot. You cannot follow the simplest instructions because you can't remember anything past the first step. You can't follow the plot of a half-hour sitcom. Your mind works at a snail's pace. You find yourself doing thirty-five miles an hour on the freeway because you cannot process the information it requires to go faster. You begin to think that you are losing your mind. You're not. You begin to think that it will always be like this. It won't.

Some people can't deal with death. At all.

Every widow I know can think of someone in her life who she thought would be there for her but wasn't. Someone who she was sure would call but didn't. That person could be a sister, a best friend, a neighbor, your mother. It's not that they don't care about you. It's just that some people cannot deal with death. They want to be there for you, but death makes them extremely uncomfortable. And now you remind them of death. Frankly, you remind everyone of death. Forgive them. They can't help it. Death is difficult, and not everyone can handle it. You don't have a choice, but they do.

The needs of the living are more important than the wishes of the dead.

It is nice to think about creating a legacy by doing something in honor of a loved one who has died, but don't let the dead dictate your life. Major decisions are best made based on the needs of the living, not the wishes of the dead.

The dead are locked in time. They don't have access to current information. They can't revise their opinions based on new experiences. At best, the desires of the dead are based on old information. Even the most opinionated person has been known to change his or her mind when circumstances change or new facts come to light.

The best way to honor deceased loved ones is to make the best decisions you can based on what you know now, not what they thought back then, when they were alive.

Everyone becomes a saint after they die.

After someone dies, any balanced reporting of that life becomes impossible. No one likes to speak ill of the dead. Unfortunately, this fact of life only works in your favor if you are the one who is dead. Everyone else is left trying to live up to this perfect person who did everything right up to the moment that he or she died.

I'm not suggesting that you go out of your way to give a balanced report on people who are no longer here to defend themselves. But it's not fair to require those of us who are still breathing to live up to an ideal that, in truth, probably never existed.

There's probably more to know about being a widow than I can tell you. But at least this is a start. Grief is a different journey for every person who undertakes it. Be brave, and don't be afraid of where it might lead you.

Insurance allows time to grieve. Make sure you have enough.

I believe that anyone in any kind of committed relationship—whether it be with a spouse, a partner, or a special friend—should strongly consider carrying life insurance. If you have children, life insurance is an absolute must. Even if you have a lot of money, you should carry some life insurance. Bank accounts, real estate, and other investments in your estate can get tied up in legal tangles that can take years to unravel; insurance pays out right away and it pays in cash. And don't worry that your loved ones will not mourn you because they will be off somewhere happily spending your insurance money. There may be instances of this happening in real life, but I don't know of any. Money can't buy happiness, but it can buy you time. An insurance payout can allow your loved ones to take the time to grieve you, without the pressure of figuring out how to pay the bills. If you buy insurance and then don't get to use it, chalk it up as the cost of living.

Get your legal stuff in order.
No excuses. Do it now.

If you don't have a will, get one. Find a lawyer *today* and make an appointment. Ask if it makes sense for you to have a trust, and if it does, then get one of those too. And while you're there, sign a power of attorney for health care decisions. All these will make it much easier on your family if you are suddenly debilitated or die. It probably won't happen, but it pays to be ready in case it does. There are books and websites that will give you more information on what you need and even help you do it yourself, but I think this is one area where it's worthwhile to buy a few hours of a lawyer's time to make sure it is done right. Don't say you'll do it next week. Do it today.

Resource
Guide

Self-Help Books

I am one of those people who think there is almost no problem that can't be helped by a trip to the bookstore. Unfortunately, in this case, I didn't find much that was very helpful.

On Death and Dying
by Elisabeth Kübler-Ross, MD
This is the book that established the famous five stages of grief—denial and isolation, anger, bargaining, depression, and acceptance. I didn't find this book helpful in dealing with grief, but it did let me learn what everyone was talking about. Just skim it.

How to Survive the Loss of a Love
by Peter McWilliams, et al
This is a gift-size book that I was given repeatedly; I wound up with five copies! I thought large parts of it were more appropriate for a teenager breaking up with her boyfriend than for an adult woman dealing with death (or divorce). But it's easy to read, and with so many short observations and quotes, chances are good you'll find at least one you like.

Widow to Widow: Thoughtful, Practical Ideas for Rebuilding Your Life
by Genevieve Davis Ginsburg, MS

This is probably one of the better self-help books. The author is a widow, but unfortunately, she writes as a therapist reporting on her patients rather than from her own experience. Still, the stories are interesting and it does contain some good tidbits of advice.

FatherLoss: How Sons of All Ages Come to Terms with the Deaths of Their Dads
by Neil Chethik

This book explores the impact of losing a father at various ages. The author does this by documenting how various well-known people dealt with their loss. I didn't find it very helpful in finding ways to help my sons cope, but I'm keeping it on my bookshelf in case they want to read it someday.

Books by Widows
First Person Singular: A Handbook for Survivors
by Lucy Miele

When a friend of my mother-in-law gave me this book just after Nick died, Lucy Miele's husband had been dead for twenty years. Yet her story compelled me because her thoughts and feelings about her husband's death were much like my own. I read it in one sitting during a sleepless night, and it was then I first realized how many parts of the widow experience are the same for everyone: The Guilties, the Angries, the Lonelies, as Mrs. Miele calls them, help to grasp the emotions of widowhood. This book is available on Amazon.com, which lists at least five books by the same title.

A Widow's Walk
by Marion Fontana

I found this book by a 9/11 widow to be a quick and interesting read. I was especially interested in seeing how she managed to comfort her son, who was only five years old when his father died. Her writing sings and her experiences ring true. Again, Amazon.com lists several books by the same title, but this one is worth looking for.

The Year of Magical Thinking
by Joan Didion

This book hardly needs a mention from me, as it is sure to become the definitive piece of serious literature on the subject of widowhood. Yet, I am amazed at how similar this famous writer's feelings and experiences are to my own. A beautifully written charting of the now-familiar (to me anyway) territory.

What Everyone Needs to Know (Because You Never Know)

No one knows what will happen to him or her today . . . or tomorrow. Here is a checklist of things that you should have. If you don't have them, get them as soon as possible.

- An up-to-date will. Make sure you sign it and get two witnesses. Keep it in a safe place and let your loved ones know where it is.

- A health care directive. This authorizes someone else to make medical decisions for you in case you can't. This form is now particularly essential because without it, a hospital will not release any information (like if you have been admitted, are in critical condition, need a transfusion, etc.) to your family members or other loved ones.

—⚹— Information on setting up a trust. A trust is simply a legal document that can help your loved ones avoid the expense of going to court to get what is rightfully theirs after you die. Not everyone needs one, but they can be extremely helpful to survivors in many situations.

—⚹— At least a minimal life insurance policy. In my opinion, there are very few people who couldn't benefit from some form of life insurance. If you think you don't need life insurance, get a minimum policy. If you know you need life insurance (like you have kids or it takes two incomes to maintain your lifestyle) get more than you think you need.

—⚹— Updated beneficiary forms. Check the beneficiary forms for your life insurance policies, retirement accounts, or other beneficiary investments regularly to make sure that they reflect your current marital situation, include all your dependents, and are in line with your wishes.

For most of the items above, it's worth enlisting the help of a professional—a lawyer, and perhaps a financial advisor. Find someone you trust. Ask friends and coworkers for recommendations, or ask at your bank. The main reason I advise you to contact a professional is that you are more likely to get everything completed—and properly signed—if you are paying someone else to do it.

Widows Online

If you insist on doing it yourself, or you at least want to get some information before you see a professional, here are some websites that may help:

WidowNet

www.widownet.org

This site was developed and is managed by a widower, Michael Goshorn, who lost his wife to cancer. He has since remarried (his wedding announcement is on the site), but he is still dedicated to keeping the site current and lively. My favorite parts of the site are *Dumb Remarks and Stupid Questions* (which made me laugh) and the wrap-up of recent articles on grief and bereavement. There are also a bulletin board and a chat room if you're into that.

Nolo

www.nolo.com

Nolo is well known for helping the average person navigate legal issues by providing books, forms, and software that are designed to be simple and understandable. Their website provides good information on wills and estate planning, in addition to family law (divorce, adoption, etc.), social security, retirement issues, and more.

Suze Orman Online

www.suzeorman.com

The diva of do-it-yourself financial planning gives very little information away for free on her website—it's mostly just her TV and personal appearance schedules. But she offers Will & Trust kits on CD for not a lot of money (well under $20) that provide all the information you need to determine if you need a trust and how much life insurance you should have. It also includes fill-in forms for making a will.

LegalZoom

www.legalzoom.com

This site, which has been featured on several major news networks, offers some free information on estate planning, but is really designed to help you create your will online for a fee, starting at about $60. That includes what they refer to as "a professional review for common mistakes." There are plenty of sites like this that offer to help you create a standard will for a fee. Just remember to get it properly signed and witnessed, and then let your loved ones know where to find it if something happens to you.

Acknowledgments

Anne Morrow Lindbergh said, "You can never repay in gratitude. You can only repay in kind somewhere else in life." There are so many people to whom I am indebted that I may not live long enough to pay it all forward.

I will never forget the kindness of those who helped me through the most difficult year of my life: Denise LaBuda, Mary Hollas, Barb and Mike Condie, Gailyn and John Johnson, Melanie DeSouza, Stephen Black, Janice DeRyss, Jim Perry, and Janice Coleman-Knight, to name a few. Thanks to the people who urged me to keep writing, especially Wendy Lichtman, Suzy Parker, Ronnie Caplane, and Greg Ellis.

This book would never have happened if not for the help and support of my friend Linda Lee Peterson. Linda got me into my first writing group, read innumerable drafts, gave invaluable comments, and kept her faith in this project, even after I had given up on it. I can't thank her enough.

Finally, thanks to my mother, who instilled in me a passion for reading and a love of words.

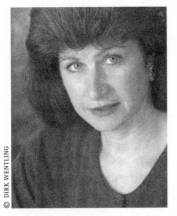

© DIRK WENTLING

About the Author

Gloria Lenhart is a marketing consultant with more than twenty-five years of experience working with companies such as Wells Fargo, Charles Schwab, Sega, and Sebastiani Vineyards. Her work has appeared in the *Chicago Tribune, Diablo Magazine,* and the *San Francisco Examiner.* An East Coast native, she lived in Washington, D.C., and Atlanta before moving to the San Francisco Bay Area in 1988. She now lives in the East Bay with her younger son, Matthew, a high school student. Her older son, Nick, is a 2005 graduate of the University of California at Davis.

Selected titles from Seal Press

For more than twenty-five years, Seal Press has published groundbreaking books. By women. For women. Visit our website at www.sealpress.com.

Literary Mama: Reading for the Maternally Inclined edited by Andrea J. Buchanan and Amy Hudock. $14.95. 1-58005-158-8. From the best of literarymama.com, this collection of personal writing includes creative nonfiction, fiction, and poetry.

Confessions of a Naughty Mommy: How I Found My Lost Libido by Heidi Raykeil. $14.95. 1-58005-157-X. The Naughty Mommy shares her bedroom woes and woo-hoos with other mamas who are rediscovering their sex lives after baby and are ready to think about it, talk about it, and *do* it.

I Wanna Be Sedated: 30 Writers on Parenting Teenagers edited by Faith Conlon and Gail Hudson. $15.95. 1-58005-127-8. With hilarious and heartfelt essays, this anthology will reassure any parent of a teenager that they are not alone in their desire to be comatose.

The Truth Behind the Mommy Wars: Who Decides What Makes a Good Mother? by Miriam Peskowitz. $15.95. 1-58005-129-4. This groundbreaking book reveals the truth behind the "wars" between working mothers and stay-at-home moms.

Solo: On Her Own Adventure edited by Susan Fox Rogers. $15.95. 1-58005-137-5. An inspiring collection of travel narratives that reveals the complexities of women journeying alone.

It's a Boy: Women Writers on Raising Sons edited by Andrea J. Buchanan. $14.95. 1-58005-145-6. Seal's edgy take on what it's really like to raise boys, from toddlers to teens and beyond.